BEDSIDE MANNA

Martin Winbolt-Lewis

Published by Martin Winbolt-Lewis

© Copyright 2013 Martin Winbolt-Lewis

ISBN 978-1-78222-061-9

Book design, layout and production management by Into Print
www.intoprint.net
+44 (0)1604 832149

Printed and bound in UK and USA by Lightning Source

'Manna' is a reference to the sticky sweet substance that sustained the wandering Israelites in the desert, as described in the Bible. Using it as the title is a not just a play on words but a reminder that holistic and spiritual care is food for people in the alien experience of ill-health.

To all my colleagues whom I have worked alongside.

CONTENTS

Contents

INTRODUCTION

"In our culture, it often seems a mark of professionalism to be impervious to another's pain. Sometimes this is a good thing: I would prefer that my surgeon operated with eyes not blurred with tears! But in many areas we have gone too far, and along with their own woundedness, our healers deny the suffering of others' suffering."

MARGARET GUENTHER (Holy Listening: The Art of Spiritual Direction)

My reason for writing this is threefold. I have been a user of the NHS for nearly 60 years, so I have observed it from the inside as a patient. Secondly, my decades in the caring professions including the 14 years as a chaplain in the NHS has taken me behind the scenes, so to speak. Finally, much of what is covered in the following pages is widely known and understood while many of its subtleties simply aren't. I feel that both for the general public who are concerned with the state of healthcare, as well as care professionals (and interested relatives and friends), my observations and insights have cried out to be recorded. My chief disclaimer is that what I have experienced has been from my own chaplaincy perspective, not a clinical one.

My first acquaintance with the NHS was at a raw age. I had an appendix operation when I was six years old. In the 1950's parents were allowed limited access to their children, and we were thus handed over to the care of others. Whether I was not told what it entailed, or I did not take it in I don't know, but I think that I was not really very well prepared for the experience. At an early stage in the proceedings I do remember being forcibly restrained in my high sided bed by a doctor with words and actions which were not very congenial to a frightened young boy of 6. I am not sure whether at the time I was resisting some procedure, hallucinating or simply that the pre-med had sent me sky high as happens sometimes, rather than having the effect of sedating me.

The only real comfort was in the fact that there was a peer group of other children going through this unpleasant experience, so at least, I was not alone. An abiding memory of that time, along with the sternness of the surroundings, the smells and the uncertainty about almost everything, was standing over the unconscious figure of a young girl, whose mouth was full of blood after her tonsillectomy. Too much exposure to reality for anyone, whether six or not! I survived though, in spite of everything.

My wife Sue had an emergency appendectomy at the more advanced age of 17. She tells her story. Upon her slow emergence from unconsciousness into the post operational world with all its disorientation and discomfort then a dawning realisation of what had happened, her eyes encountered what she thought was the Grim Reaper in person. A dark figure was bent over her recumbent body. The large white clerical collar was matched by a set of prominent white teeth, framed by a thatch of equally white hair. This apparition belonged to a rotund clergyman, presumably a chaplain, who spoke some *bon mot* into her ear which was understandably lost on her. He then left. She did however, for a moment think her time had come.

Thankfully not all first experiences of healthcare are like this!

Bedside Manna has been written to highlight the fact that the manner of bedside approaches has to take into consideration the fact that although the NHS is brilliant in many ways, increasingly there are bits missing too. My time in the NHS as a chaplain spent listening to countless thousands tells me that it has not really grasped that it is both a relief and scary for people to be ill or in hospital. To the very young, the elderly and confused as well as those with learning disabilities good, warm communication is so very vital. When things go wrong, as they do from time to time, taking the people very seriously and admitting it in a human way, will bring much less in the way of litigation than the arms-length bureaucratic approach that can prevail and so riles people. This bedside manner is especially necessary in the way we deal with anxious and bereaved relatives. How we are treated matters so much. At those moments we are far less interested in procedures that have been followed, than human understanding and kindness. The quality of relationships made and experienced in healthcare should be a priority today, because the way which we are clinically treated for the most part is excellent as thousands of patients make a habit of telling me. How we come over to people when they are

8

vulnerable is actually a vital part of the healing process. The question is whether that is recognised universally.

As an 'accidental' researcher over several years I have had the privilege of observing the patient experience at close quarters in a capacity that perhaps no other health care professional can. Many of the insights and choice of anecdotes stem from this observation and listening. When thousands of patients repeatedly tell you the same kind of things, you have to take notice. These insights and reflections on sickness and its collateral damage may be helpful for doctors and nurses, as well as health care professionals, faith representatives and church workers; anyone in fact who is interested in patient care or cares for a long term sick relative.

The World Health Organisation recognises that health is about "a dynamic state of complete physical, spiritual and social well- being and not merely the absence of disease and infirmity" (1) It is the spiritual, or those things which impact most on the essence and meaning of our humanness, that need to be recognised and addressed within the health care setting. The deeper aspects of living are as essential to a person's total well- being and can often add to a person's sense of self-worth and powers of recovery and resilience. Holistic and spiritual factors can add a bonus dimension beyond a physical recovery alone. They allow us to reflect on what is going on inside us as we meet the turbulence surrounding the challenge to our well -being that accompanies illness.

1

SETTING THE SCENE

It is usually helpful to know why a book is being written. "Bedside Manna" has been a slow growing product deriving from of over fourteen years of spending a large proportion of each working day listening to sick and traumatised people and trying to support them. It is as a result of these experiences that I personally feel that there is a need to share what I have discovered through these encounters. They form a coherent pattern which suggests patients need to express something of their inner world in those circumstances which are so challenging to face. I also believe we are at a crucial stage in the history of the NHS, where the monastic and military influences - pastoral and organisational - which have helped to form modern healthcare are slowly being eroded and are replaced with a more medical, mechanistic and scientific, business led approach. The result has been that the pastoral side of medicine is being superseded by the 'medical model'. This is primarily about diagnosis through tests and then fixing the problem. I hope I am not being unfair to a very committed group of health professions. The pastoral and clinical dimensions of healthcare should be collaborative, but with budgets pressured, they have to compete; with the clinical (probably understandably) winning hands down. Perhaps now we need to challenge the Health Service in the name of a deeper quality of engagement with the patient in the interests of total health. Well- being is much more than being well.

Over the past decade the National Health Service has found itself the subject of analysis, comment and enquiry in the media on a daily basis. Much of this is sadly negative. The Patients Charter of 1991 attempted to put more power into the hands of patients. In the years following their elevation to power in 1997, the Labour Government had tried to pour much needed resources, human and financial into the Health Service. Somehow the fruits of this provision have not been easy to assess, as the institution has been under pressure for a long time. The NHS Plan which found flesh in Your Guide to the NHS (2001) which states "NHS Staff will respect your privacy and dignity. They will be sensitive to, and respect, your religious, spiritual and cultural needs at all times."(2) In latter improvements consumers and the public have been given input into service configurations and changes in service delivery. In addition Government targets have been given in areas ranging from Accident and Emergency 'turnaround' times, to designated targets for cancer, outpatient treatments and surgery. In spite of so much attention, the National Health Service is generally seen to be struggling with the twin burdens of governmental pressures on the one hand and the renewed public expectation that further funding has brought about. Nursing staff end up as the filler in this 'sandwich'. The present Coalition Government of 2010 is now seriously looking at a reform of the NHS, though the NHS Future Forum, asked to review its implications, have advised against over emphasis on competition, and warned against the role of the private sector in health. 'Constant change is here to stay' has been the NHS motto for a while now, and everyone involved has felt the strain of that constant change. No wonder there is so much potential for strained relationships of all kinds both on the wards and in the Trust HQ's, both with nursing staff, middle management and patients.

CHALLENGING THE IMPERSONAL

Along with these rigorous attempts to improve patient flow and efficiency and deliver better performance for them, the last few years have witnessed an approach to patient care that personally reminds me more of industrial and commercial efficiency initiatives than what should constitute the delicate treatment of vulnerable persons whatever rhetoric is used. Under these conditions there is a great temptation for health professionals to treat patients as units to be mended rather than persons to be given concerned hospitality, focused attention and expertise. Max Pemberton, doctor and columnist wrote recently in the Daily Telegraph about reforms in the Health Service, "Competition in the health service does not work. It drives down the cost of procedures but, with it, quality too.

It emphasises profits over patients." In so describing the dangers he also comments " No longer the National Health service, but NHS plc. a brand name; nothing more." (3) This is a particularly important insight because in this unique institution people have to struggle with one of the most underrated and difficult experiences in life, that of being ill or hospitalised. At the risk of blowing the issue out of proportion, I believe that my thousands of encounters with patients and their stories tell me that they did find a sense of trauma in their experience of illness and hospitalisation. I know people react differently. Some are very stoic, some very supported and resilient, but I would hold my ground on this one. This growing de-personalising of the health care experience goes hand in hand now with a language that extols the *patient experience* as the most important feature in health care delivery. It does little to lessen the trauma.

Whilst nothing but the improvement in the quality of health services is desired by politicians and Hospital Trust Boards, the reality of the actual patient's emotional experience is now more often that of living through a kind of 'biological garage' whilst in hospital. As the Bishop of St Albans, the recent Chair of the Hospitals Chaplaincies Council said in a speech in February 2007 during the Second Reading of the Palliative Care Bill, "Language is always significant, and if we use only mechanistic language to shape our thinking about palliative care, we shall end up treating human beings like robots. This same kind of mechanistic, detached language which is widely used in the NHS, is seeking to explain our NHS rationale of treating people. Is this a dangerous signal about how the NHS truly views human beings?" (4) In a similar vein recently the head of the Trades Union Unison warned against viewing patients as *customers*. Karen Jennings said "The concern that I have is the term customer. What we are hearing more and more is the application of business ethos in the NHS. Equating patients with consumers is not useful." One may ask what set of values that relate to fellow human beings does the NHS follow and which govern this approach?

Jennings continues; "When you come into the health service you are very vulnerable. You rely on the expertise and knowledge and skills of the staff that are going to deliver that service. It's about how you approach the people you are looking after and that has nothing to do with being a customer."(5)   From following this approach to people how do we keep in focus the fact that sick people are a fragile community. Their ultimate worth and value desperately requires institutional recognition, especially in this all important health care setting? How can appropriate institutional care be given, if the NHS itself does not really feel the *level of trauma* and anxiety that sickness and accident brings to the lives of the countless millions passing through its doors? All this mirrors the cyber processes that pervade all of our contemporary life, where computers seem to handle a great deal of administration, and where joined up thinking is often a rare luxury. We are fast becoming the "Computer says No" generation, where common sense and interpersonal intricacies are simply not high on the agenda. So much attention is given to the cognitive functioning relating to keyboard skills required today, that we are apt to forget the human side in our transactions. The human psyche is more complicated than our electronics! From my experience the NHS does not resist this trend. All very well you may think, it speeds up the once laborious paper processes in all walks of life; but when things go wrong as regularly happens, the voices behind the Call Centre monitors that handle our query, are not always the ones with any real care for the frustration going on for the customers. Perish the thought that healthcare should go the same way.

2

CHANGES IN THE CULTURAL CLIMATE

Economic, social and philosophical changes over the last two hundred years have also had their effect over how we view people as they go through health problems. Sociologically we have moved away from of the agrarian world of dependence upon rain and sun for subsistence. Through massive industrialisation and population growth and a migration from the land into the cities we have evolved as a society that depends more on the appliance of science and technology than the fickleness of nature or, as some may imagine, God. However, in the same way as appeals were once made to fertility rites or appeals to religious leaders in rural and agricultural economies in many matters, we now appeal to a technocracy in our post- industrial, technologically dependent society. In our making any appeal to technical experts, we will then refer back to scientific knowledge and method. Research findings and 'evidence based practice' is today's clarion call in this regard. We hear it all the time in healthcare. However as Cristina Odone, no stranger to the intricacies of long term health care, wrote in regard to her brother's Lorenzo's situation brought to prominence in the film "Lorenzo's Oil", " Scientific progress is not just about academic laurels, but about real people."(6)

Today we are responsible for running society efficiently, including matters of healthcare. Today it is achieved with a greater and greater appeal to technical expertise. There is nothing wrong in that. We attempt to manage people and resources in this way rationally using our heads but subtly bypassing a complementary dependence upon the experiential knowledge of the past. This is all of course in the interests of material progress, economic prosperity and control over our environment. In a climate that promotes this predominantly rational and academic approach perhaps other deeper, more spiritual values have been neglected with de-personalising results. Healthcare, which is primarily about *persons* is a prime casualty.

Robin Youngson writing in a NHS Confederation Future Debates paper written in 2008 has commented: "In the meantime as nursing practice extends farther into the previous domains of medical practice there is increasing tension between evidence-based nursing care with its scientific research agenda, and broader policy directions for nursing with a holistic concern for the whole patient."(7)

EVIDENCE AND EMPATHY

Whilst clearly vital in many areas such as the diagnostic and patterns of treatment, research led and 'proven' outcomes have overshadowed the more intuitive and the pastoral approaches of the past. In the quality of relationships that is required in care, no amount of research can replace basic common sense. We *know* hurting people require an empathetic approach. Perhaps that is why the vulnerable in society have always needed someone to fight their cause. Hard factual evidence is what many decisions in healthcare and social provision are based upon, and rightly so. However it is not right that what cannot conform to this approach is to lose status as acceptable reality. As the Church of England has identified in its recent 2009 guidelines for working with people with learning disabilities and those on the autistic spectrum, there can be an overemphasis upon the role of intellect and rationality in the world of faith. This tends to marginalise those less able to access this dimension of life. The same is so with healthcare, for along with the research led and intellectual approaches should come the intuitive and empathetic dimensions also. If a person is troubled you respond. You don't need a research project to decide whether you should. Today, however skilled and competent medical care may be, the human spirit cannot be dismissed as not of prime interest to health professionals without injury to the people concerned. As Charles Davis comments about the society of the day with its highly materialistic preoccupations in the 1970's; "Thus consciousness is contracted in a way that excludes the spiritual and the transcendent from reality."(8) Illness has a habit of teasing out the fact that we are not one dimensional human beings; a lot goes on beneath the surface.

With this drift, such aspects of care such as compassion and empathy, intuition and the wisdom of experience are in danger of being marginalised to what is an evidence based culture. When budget cuts are made, chaplaincies are often the first to feel their effects. In Worcester in 2006, chaplaincy was cut to its barest minimum engendering a public outcry. People do matter, which is why a chaplaincy which provides an empathetic presence amid the other time-constricted professions is so important. It is as if we as a society and within the NHS have lost confidence in what previous generations have valued, the recognition of the whole person, not just the bits that malfunction. Perhaps it is because these things are harder to justify intellectually and financially in the climate of today. The era of the shaman and the village elders has disappeared, but I believe we need the modern equivalent.

Chris Swift, a past College of Healthcare Chaplains President draws attention to the risks that emerge from negating the deeper needs patients may have on purely budgetary grounds. "Within health care chaplaincy, the latest and most significant sign of disregard for the vulnerable comes with the quiet falling apart of our out-of-hours on call. Despite the prosperity of society, the billions spent on the NHS under New Labour, an inexpensive and compassionate system of care for those at the end of life is vanishing. The total market has crept into the side rooms of our hospitals and made its presence felt." **(9)**

It needs to be said in defence of the thoroughness of research, evidence-based practice and meticulous paperwork covering our every intervention and the highly bureaucratic hinterland of healthcare today, that constant litigation has required a higher degree of responsibility in the NHS requiring paperwork to back up most interventions. To put it bluntly you have to cover your back. You simply cannot tell what will end up in a court of law these days! The procedures, policies and protocols we follow have to be shown to be safe and responsible. The recognition of human value and its sensitive treatment in ill health have as much currency today as it ever did. This is why the place of open-ended support in hospitals which can give time, interest and empathetic care is so vital to preserve *as a healing factor*. Admirable and effective though much of the reliance on research and evidence based practice may be, it may be foolish to ignore other complementary approaches. This is especially true of the intuitive and interactive world of human engagement. Some years ago my father was extremely ill in hospital but none of the clinicians were able to put a finger on what caused his high temperatures. It took two weeks and his decline to refer him to another consultant in another hospital. It was the right move. The consultant in question examined him, asked some questions and pronounced, "Oh, I know this one, I think it's sub- acute endocarditis," and it was. He was then treated effectively because the consultant in question had *experience* of that condition, so that he *knew* immediately. It bears out the old Chinese proverb; *I hear; I forget. I see: I understand. I do: I remember.*

3

RESTORING TRIED PATHS OF CARE

In the light of this present climate I believe that we need to restore this forgotten heart of care to the NHS. This heart is all about holistic and spiritual care as expressed in compassion. Compassion literally means *suffering with,* a capacity demonstrated through a concern for the whole person. "A closed heart lacks compassion." is the observation of Marcus Borg who continues;" In the Bible compassion portrayed as the ability to feel the feelings of another at a lower level than one's head, "in the womb", "in the bowels" and to act accordingly. A closed heart does not feel this. Though it can be charitable, it does not feel the suffering of others."(10) Alongside all these welcomed NHS efficiencies such as performance targets as well as the careful oversight of resources, allied with many technological and procedural innovations and pharmaceutical research, I believe that the NHS needs to also provide for the *actual trauma* that accompanies ill-health and accident.

Once this particular insight is recognised as of prime importance to health, it should be reflected by a budgetary consideration. The Studer Group, an outcomes based consulting firm in healthcare have researched the aspect of attentive concern for patient welfare and concluded that patients are more contented and less liable to press their buzzers for attention when this happens. (11) It may require a greater share of scarce resources but maybe those resources might be cost effective in the long run. A service with empathy as well as clinical excellence is no bad target to aim for. Our patients are vulnerable people who are in transit through our hospitals, hospices and clinics and many will progress into our operating theatres and beds. Alongside state of the art excellence, a certain sentience is also required. We need the ability that sees that a temperature check on their human fragility might also be part of integrated care.

"Hey, that's *my* body!"

Having experienced a major operation recently I have had the experience of finding the good and the not so good in the NHS. Despite all the unquestionably excellent things that were done for me during my five day stay, I was also left with the feeling that my aftercare was not very good. It was when I left the 'womb' of the hospital that my anxieties began to surface. At home I had no one to answer my questions. I was not warned about the disconcerting things that would happen to my body whilst in immediate recovery, or the feelings that would accompany these things. Often I find that this angst occurs in the small hours of the morning. I felt very alone. In the ward I was getting the best of attention. The job was not done so well in the follow up. I felt I needed more thorough preparation for my recovery. As a human being with feelings however, who was having to deal with new and sometimes alarming physical and emotional experiences that were never addressed, I was not being treated *holistically*. In my hospital stay no one ever asked how I was *feeling*. It felt to me like only a part of me was being mended. I was not an impassive bystander in it all. Using these kinds of insights during my own hospitalisation has been all important in the development of my role as a chaplain, so I suppose that there was a plus side to the whole experience.

This shortfall of care in my opinion was largely due to the fact that I was not properly *prepared* for what might happen once I left the security of the hospital. In fairness, it could be argued that few, if any, of the staff had actually been through the operation themselves, so how could they know? Maybe I was wrong to expect too much empathy. Both at moments during my stay in the ward and more especially when I went home in my more desperate moments, I actually felt a measure of neglect not medically but holistically. Upon reaching by specially adapted bedroom when I returned home I surprised myself by suddenly bursting into tears. I can only think it was the trauma surfacing.

I see now that I could not have anticipated this strange twilight world of recovery. As things progressed the more I got into my recovery and rehabilitation from hip surgery, the less joined up I found the thinking on aftercare. Neither the hospital, the local Social Services nor my G.P. Practice wanted to give me the aids I needed, such as an elevated toilet seat, chair raisers and a "grabber" to save me bending down. I "borrowed" them in the end from the Occupational Therapy Department where I worked! I wondered about those people with no helpful backup like mine? Also I found the advice on how long I should use my crutches varied. I had to ask around among friends who had also had the same procedure. Everyone I asked seemed to come up with something different; the hospital, a physiotherapist friend, my G.P. and the surgeon who operated on me. Weighing up all this advice, I ended up by discarding them. It worked. If an important aspect of our spiritual need (see Chapter 2; Spiritual Needs) addresses the *quality* of the communication between health professionals and patients undergoing the disorientation of ill health I certainly had a *nul points* experience!

4

THE HUMANITARIAN TASK

A question this book does seek to address is about identifying some of the traumas associated with ill health and hospitalisation and what constitutes good holistic and spiritual care in the situation. We might also ask "who provides it?" I will try to deal with how spiritual care can be exercised without causing further burnout to those concerned, leaving them short of resources to do their "day job". The answers to these questions as we shall discover are far from complex. They are about being the human beings we are, and developing awareness of what is going on in the people we encounter.

The first theme that regularly crops up is that we tend to *underestimate* the emotional trauma of being hospitalised. If we simply acknowledge this one fact it really helps. Whether we are clinicians or members of the support staff we can become so over familiar with all that we do in our professional life that we run the risk of failing to "see" the *person* in the patient. Secondly, the function of "holistic" and "spiritual" care is to allow our own humanity to engage with the human being in front of us in the hospital bed. I read a logo somewhere in the hospital recently; "we think as professionals, but we act as human beings." This bold assertion is one we have to carry in our minds humbly and ask of ourselves every day when dealing with vulnerable people. Do we manage it all the time; probably not, being human ourselves?

Perhaps, the most effective thing we can do, and most people are able to this to one degree or another, is simply to be *present* to patients as one fellow human being to another, to actively listen to their concerns, expressed verbally or otherwise. This simple approach often helps them to know that they are not alone in going through this difficult experience of ill health. My plea in this book is that we might try to put ourselves in their place. After all, none of us knows when we might exchange places with them. Health, after all, is such a precious and fragile thing. The National Institute for Clinical Excellence Guidance on Cancer Services has also identified the de-stabilising effects of ill health. Illness and accident can have devastating effects on both a patient's life and their family. This is something we shall be looking at later. It undermines self- worth, and throws up all sorts of questions. We define ourselves by our wellness, and it is hard to think of our identity the same way when sick. Lance Armstrong, the American seven times winner of the Tour de France (and now discredited over serious doping during those years) articulates the problem "Cancer would change everything for me. It just wouldn't derail my career. It would deprive me of my entire definition of who I was. Who could I be if I could no longer be myself, the person I used to know? A sick person"(12)

5

WHAT ON EARTH IS SPIRITUAL CARE?

To begin with we might ask, "where does spiritual care fit in to health care?" The answer lies within the integrated dimensions of care in the NHS. There are many levels of care, which are complementary and often collaborative. Medical staff will view the patient from the point of the 'illness' and ask questions, do tests, take samples and discover from the signs and symptoms the causation and pathology of a condition. This will lead to diagnosis and treatment. On this next stage of the journey the nursing staff will attend to supporting and caring for the patient, and doing some of the administration of drugs and medicines' as time goes on, certainly where rehabilitation is required, others in the therapies (Occupational, physiotherapy, dietetics, speech therapy, clinical psychology) will assist recovery, both physically and psychologically.

Patients may well have their philosophy of life challenged from what has happened to them. This will be dealt with later in this book. They may find they have to grapple with issues of anxiety, alienation, meaning, loss and just not feeling at home with things generally. Spiritual care concerns itself with all this as well as notions of failure, guilt, right and wrong, even death or a sense of God or the ultimate meaning of things. Spiritual care may or may not include the meeting of religious needs, which the NHS considers an important part of equality and diversity. For Muslims particularly, religious considerations make a lot of difference to the degree to which they might feel at ease in hospital.

The term *spiritual care* is spoken of repeatedly in this book. Some people will have an idea about what it means, many won't. It will sound rather mystical and grand to some, even spooky, whilst others will have a vague idea that spirituality is about meaning and purpose and those directions and values in life that we as human beings carry in our inner being. Spiritual issues are not necessarily religious, but could be, and therefore are in the public domain. We may not wish to talk about deep things at social gatherings, but when life deals us a blow, or devastating events happen to us, we may drop our defences and air some of our assumptions about the way the world is and what as human beings we reach out for in life.

At the simplest level we could say spiritual care is discovering and nurturing that which enlivens a person. This may range from family to faith, from holidays to sport. Having led a varied life, I found much of my background being used to take part in the discussions of others' interests. I remember coming across a woman who looked rather like a ghost. It was afternoon, and she was in the next bed that I was coming across. We chatted and in her lethargic state, awaiting an operation and clearly not well, she mentioned something about classical music. Although as my wife will tell you, I am a graduate of the school of bluff, I do have a passing understanding and appreciation of classical music. Once we started talking about composers, musical pieces, orchestras and venues she started to come alive. When I left some twenty minutes later she was positively buzzing. She had become awake because a passion in her life had been recognised and affirmed; she was no longer just a patient in a hospital bed.

Definitions of spirituality and therefore spiritual care do exist, but none captures the whole of the complex world it embraces the same way as the word 'love' can mean many things in different contexts. That does not mean that we should not try to shed light upon it. Murray and Zentner describe the spiritual in a 1989 nursing paper as: "A quality that goes beyond religious affiliation. That strives for aspirations, reverence, awe, meaning and purpose, even in those who do not believe in any god." (13)

HELPFUL DEFINITIONS

A helpful definition can also be found in work by Johnston and Mayers. "Spirituality can be defined as the search for meaning and purpose in life which may or may not be related to a belief in God, or some form of higher power. For those with no conception of supernatural belief, spirituality may relate to the notion of a motivating life force, which includes an integration of the dimensions of mind, body and spirit. This personal belief or faith also shapes a person's perspective on the world and is expressed in the way he/she lives life. Therefore spirituality is experienced through connectedness to God/higher being, and/or by one's relationships with self, others or nature." **(14)**

I am not wishing to downplay religion as opposed to spirituality. Both are very important for people, but sometimes people have a spiritual side yet for reasons of their own steer clear of religious expression or belief, or indeed organised religion. There is enough evidence to suggest however that a faith that is part of a person's life helps in a time of difficulty. Dr Raj Persaud commenting in a newspaper article about research undertaken in the United States by Dr M. McCullough on religion and health points out that; "Religion appears to bestow on believers a contentment and resilience in the face of misfortune that is due to the hope provided by faith, with which modern medicine and psychotherapy can still, even after thousands of years, simply not compete." **(15)** This positive view of the sense of meaning that religion can (but it is not guaranteed) provide is highlighted by Koenig and Larsen; "When people become physically ill, many rely on religious beliefs and practices to relieve stress, retain a sense of control, and maintain hope and their sense of meaning and purpose in life. Religious involvement appears to enable the sick, particularly those with serious and disabling medical illness, to cope better and experience psychological growth from their negative health experiences, rather than being defeated or overcome by them." **(16)** In another piece of research in 2001 by Koenig, McCullough and Larson it was concluded that the benefit of religion and spirituality to health and well- being are threefold - it aids prevention, speeds recovery and foster composure in the face of ill health. Basically to have a framework of faith beyond the material does aid resilience.

I think personally of the example of Joni Eareckson Tada who dived into a lake at 16 and hit a rock and broke her neck, thus rendering her paraplegic. From being a healthy girl she became catapulted into a world of intensive rehabilitation, depression, questioning and huge readjustment. Staggeringly, her traumatic accident eventually led her to encourage others, and she learned to draw, sing and write and speak publicly. She was for me personally, a great inspiration for many years. Unique as she was as a person, it has to be said that it was her faith that gave her life meaning even if Plan A had to be torn up and consigned to the rubbish bin.

Kathy Galloway says; "For after all what is our spirituality other than our profoundest motivations, our deepest desires, those longings, instincts, intuitions, insights and dreams, which animate us, breathe through us, move us and inspire us, and which we value and prioritise according to our cultural conditioning, our belief systems and out life experience and concerns."(17)

I hope some light has been shed on a subject that is not easy to pinpoint. The fact is that many people undergoing the swings and roundabouts of illness and accident find the experience distressing. To heed these things becomes *value added*, as many have testified through the thank-you letters our department receives every year.

6

SPIRITUAL NEEDS

Spiritual distress is a present factor in illness and hospitalisation. Some research done by a colleague of mine, Roger Cressey, with help from the Palliative Care Team of doctors, chaplains and a counsellor in the 1990s identified the key issues which had a bearing on this experience of this distress, and they seemed to cluster around a set of needs that people had in hospital, and which, if not met, created anxiety and a feeling of being vulnerable and alienated. The list, which was pared down from a broad 150 to a convenient 10 were as follows:

Being valued
Finding meaning
Having hope
Emotions
Having dignity
Truth and honesty
Good communication
Death, dying, bereavement and loss
Religion
Culture.(18)

If we think about this list and the categories outlined, I think we might all be aware of those dimensions that form part of all our basic needs in living creatively. They can provide a congenial atmosphere for trying to find a peaceful centre within oneself in an often bewildering world. In other words *everyone has spiritual needs*. Translated into language we may all use, it is about whom we are and what our lives may be all about. These needs require careful addressing in hospital to keep us in touch with ourselves.

To offer spiritual care is to recognise people have human value and depth and that things matter when you are ill or in hospital. It offers space for people to go there if they choose to. Spiritual care is never invasive but tries to be supportive, empathetic and compassionate. It can be practical as well as emotionally helpful. As a challenge to the direction in which healthcare has moved, to think that we can ignore the non- physical aspects of a patient's life, which are either precious to them or resulting in their emotional or spiritual distress, is to totally misunderstand the breadth of the word 'healing'. I really do not think we can use the term 'healing' for health care which knowingly denies these dimensions of a person's life.

Nursing perspectives and a case in point

Wilf McSherry has done much valuable work on the nursing perception of the spiritual aspects of healthcare. The general nursing position he drew from his work was that they recognised a patient's religion or spirituality was very important to them, and that they needed support in this area. In general they found it hard to define exactly what this meant, and felt inadequate to provide this aspect of care themselves. This work in their opinion was to be devolved to chaplains, but chaplains often say we are all a part of the workforce who *could* offer this One of his conclusions, interestingly enough was that "Nurses perceive spirituality as a universal concept which they feel is relevant to all individuals."(19)

I have seen often enough the devastating results of illness upon people over the years. In the 60,000-70,000 visits I have made to the bedside, either randomly as 'blanket visiting' or by referral, I have observed how much more readily people are prepared to talk than in the wellness of everyday life. Many would disclose something of their deeper selves in their vulnerable state that accompanies a stay in hospital. Doris met a crossroads in her life when she found herself in the *same ward* as her daughter who had died there. The staff were very apologetic, but said that it was the only bed available. When I came across her on a routine visit she explained this. At the time she was shaken to the core and did not know how she was going to cope with it.

Her daughter's death had, in her own words, "cast a shadow over her life" which was then compounded by her husband's death three years ago. Every morning she described a feeling of dread when she woke up. Though each day was different, she felt nothing "was ever right again" since her daughter's death. Now she was repeating her daughter's experience, or so it seemed. Spiritual distress? I should certainly say so.

Amazingly though, far from being the traumatic experience she feared, this carbon copy of her daughter's last journey had actually had the most positive and healing outcome. The nursing staff had been kind and sensitive to her, and she felt loved within this ward that she most feared entering. In the quiet and stillness of treatment and bed rest, *something lifted.* She felt a deep healing that she couldn't explain. In her words she felt that she needed "to go back into her daughter's experience" to somehow "know that it was all right." The upshot for Doris was a release from the feelings of fear, anxiety and depression. The ward had become for her a place of reconciliation with a traumatic past.

The icing on the cake for her was to be able to then explain this to a chaplain who would not laugh at her but value the experience that she had gone through. Despite all she had gone through Doris wanted to shout her new found peace of mind from the rooftops. For her the aspect of spiritual care that mattered was the ability to speak of things to someone else who would understand, in order to complete the circle. It happened to be a chaplain. It could have been someone else!

I never met Doris again. I don't know how particularly spiritual she was in her everyday life. What happened that day however meant something and tapped into a deep part of her life.

Perhaps we should allow Her Majesty Queen Elizabeth to have the last word on this subject from her Christmas Day speech in 2000: "Whether we believe in God or not, I think most of us have a sense of the spiritual, the recognition of a deeper meaning and purpose in our lives." Doris certainly recognised that!

7

THE TRAUMA OF INTERRUPTED LIVING

"I don't feel myself today". How often have we said that or heard something similar? Ill health tends to take away a person's place in the community. It has a profound effect on people, who find themselves sidelined by their inability to do ordinary things like maintaining relationships and enjoying pleasures. As a socially grey area, sickness can affect others as they relate to the sick person. The normal providers of self-esteem like work, achievement, positive relationships and recreations cannot function so well for the unwell and the person is often left a shadow of their former self during bad health. It is interesting to note that in the healing stories of Jesus in the Gospels, healing was often aimed at two levels. The first was the immediate need and that was physical, but the second, more subtle healing was the restoring of that sick person's place in society. In those days and that culture many illnesses were considered to be some God inspired punishment that merited social exclusion. This was particularly true of leprosy. In the healing described in Mark's Gospel **(20)**, once the physical cure was made the leper was told by Jesus to show his healing to the priest who would effectively see evidence of his right to enter society again. You might say in today's terms, the priest's affirming of real healing was the evidence-base that society required for social inclusion after bearing the stigma of leprosy. He couldn't get involved in the structures of life.

There can be a feeling amongst the unwell when everyone around you is getting on with life that illness equals a kind social redundancy. In their paper of Spiritual Care giving in Nursing Practice, Price, Stevens and Labarre say that " illness is demeaning in Western Culture, which prizes youth and vitality, and so the challenge to find self- worth during sickness is all the more difficult."**(21)**

INTERRUPTED RELATIONSHIPS

Sickness may be found to steal your place in life. The trauma of becoming ill marks a break in the continuity of existence, and a change can occur in a person's sense of self. Marion was in an orthopaedic ward. She was an elderly lady who had recently fallen and broken her leg. Dignified and thoughtful, Marion couldn't help shedding a tear as she described what this latest accident had done to her.

Although she had been widowed for over a decade, she had a supportive family and a wonderful group of friends. These long-term friends formed a group that met several times a year for outings and holidays. They were her 'rock' in life, as she described them. The timing of her recent fall could not have been worse. It had happened just before one of these holidays they had planned together. The holiday was booked, and they had made final arrangements. Her friends were all so understanding, and stressed to Marion that they would be happy to cancel, but selflessly she persisted in making them continue with it.

Marion was apologetic to me as she broke down in tears. She cried for a few moments and continued to speak. She explained how she had a skin graft a year or two ago, and that she "had been strong and stood up to all that". This time, however she felt that she was not so strong. The main factor in this is that she became vulnerable, thinking that her friends would be cementing their relationships and having fun while she was immobile and feeling helpless. She was also wondering whether she would ever go on any of these friendship holidays again.

So Marion's life was affected by her present incapacity. At the time she could not see beyond it. Her condition had the effect of diminishing her as a person. It is this kind of encounter in hospital that will strike the healthcare professional or regular visitor to patients as difficult and sad. As Marion temporarily lost her place in the community, so others find their experiences to be similar.

I remember well how on another occasion a man talked proudly of the new Mercedes car that be had bought, but how it was standing idle in the garage. There was a certain wistfulness in him as he realised that the dreams he had fulfilled had been put on hold because he would not be able to drive for a long time. Whoever we are in the community,

31

homeless, duchess or even politician, sickness has this capacity to level us. Other than being treated privately we all have to wait out turn for diagnosis, tests and treatment. This can make us feel less than the person we believe ourselves to be. There are usually no favours granted because *you* are socially more secure than the person opposite you. For some people that is not an easy experience to live with.

In these ways hospital admission and treatment, particularly if we are feeling very ill at the time, bring people startlingly into the immediate present with all its insecurities. The past and even the future sometimes become pale and distant realities.

ILLNESS CAN ALTER SOCIAL DYNAMICS

Illness and hospitalisation may also hijack your relationships. Family and friends are very much part of the fabric of most peoples' lives. They help us define who we are, they help us develop as people and they nurture and support us at times when we most need them. I would be accused of a lack of realism if I did not say that occasionally relationships can also be challenging, selfish and abusive and sometimes drive us mad. I would like to think that families and friends come out more strongly on the 'plus' side for most of us in our hour of need, thus creating a safe place in a world which can at times feel hostile.

When people have accidents, become sick or need surgery, the nature of these close relationships may be seen to change according to what is happening. Some patients I have encountered (admittedly some have been rather confused) have felt that their families want them to die because they are after their money. I have to say that when people enter a paranoid phase this frequently happens. I do not doubt that in some instances this is exactly the regrettable circumstance that some ill people meet.

I have also met people in tears, so worried by the fact that their children as mature adults, would literally not 'let them go'. Several of these people have been very ill, weary and just want to die quietly, but they fear the overzealous efforts of their family in keeping them around to meet their agendas however worthy. Often this is because the relatives are fearful of loss, which is understandable. Sometimes it is because they still need that person very badly, and fear to go on living without their presence in their lives. I remember praying with one woman who asked for me to do this whilst her family were there in order to bring about some kind of 'closure'. She wanted permission from those dearest to her to die. Everyone, it seems used the moment to 'let go'. Surprisingly, she was out of hospital within a few days! It must have been a truly healing moment when her family let go of her. They actually got her back with interest!

I can remember another moment when I was called out in the early hours to a lady who knew she was dying. I read to her from the Bible as she requested and said some prayers. She was so comforted by what she heard that she insisted I stayed another hour until her daughters arrived. She was not a particularly religious person however, but she wanted to get a few things off her chest and had asked for a chaplain. When her daughters turned up, it felt as if all this good work of preparation was destroyed as they tearfully pleaded with her not to be so 'morbid'. It appears she was ready for the beyond; they were not. It was hard watching this. In the end, the lady knew best because she died very quickly, and the family dynamics had to adjust to the inevitable.

Relationships are generally challenged when people experience life changing accidents or conditions such as spinal injuries, strokes and brain haemorrhages. In these scenarios the person's life changes out of all recognition at a stroke (excuse the pun). Sometimes this can happen in a flash, as in a road accident or a stroke. There is no time to take it in. The adjustment here is traumatic for all concerned. The person's loved ones often remain in shock and cannot accept what is happening around them. What often happens in these situations is that the person and their family and friends have to draw a line under 'how it was', and start again. Many spinal injury patients have told me that ' you just have to get on with it.' They have gradually realised that life will never return to how it was. A new start for everyone is needed. This has an effect on relationships. Some marriages founder on the 'bridge too far' of this need to adjust.

REALITY CHECKS

In our Spinal Injuries Unit certainly, a hospital myth circulates about marriage breakdown after spinal injuries. People will put it down to the long term effects of this kind of trauma. I have seen young people whose partner has gone on to marry them whilst knowing they would never have a "normal" relationship. Is it guilt? Is it the desire to make it all better for the patient? I don't honestly know, but it takes a lot of courage and commitment for the marriage to last and grow. So often the dreams that most couples have are shattered in a split second. Another cause of spinal injury apart from traumatic accident is neurosurgery that does not work out as hoped for. After initial committed support and understanding, a realisation of how life might be in the future gradually dawns on the able bodied partner. As the shock of the trauma fades so sometimes does the desire to go on with the relationship. It is sad but it happens.

One other myth I have heard is that the partner of a spinally injured person is faced by the clinicians with the challenge to review whether they want to go on with the relationship fairly immediately after injury. The argument went that for the patient another loss or adjustment is thrown into the general pool of 'things to cope with', and that it is kinder to do the hard thing sooner than later when hopes of permanence in the relationship may have built up.

In the way I have described it this kind of challenge may sound cold and unfeeling. Perhaps the accumulated experience of clinicians has led them to the conclusion that a short and sharp severance is actually less painful in the long run. It does not sound good either way, but how many of us have been faced with that kind of painful decision? I wonder what we might do in a similar situation?

In general terms any relationship may be strained when a family has to commit itself to an open-ended routine of visiting. Having recently had a hip replacement, I saw my wife every day as she drove a considerable way to support me. It was wonderful and I am very grateful. I did tell her not to come every day, but I am glad she did. Many patients do the same, especially if their partner is elderly or has to catch three buses to get to the hospital. However, I was only in

34

for the best part of five days. That is totally different from those who spend months, even years, in rehabilitation. Illness alters relationships in many ways. Wonderfully, some deepen and show great commitment and care, but it is not always so. Whichever way it turns it is a painful reality check.

8

COMPASSION FATIGUE; WALKING THAT MILE TOO FAR

In these days of high expectation in our health service, repeated Government intervention in its workings, and a shrinking pot of money that hardly keeps pace with mounting pressures on health provision, it is hardly surprising that something might give. The media regularly tells us that. Stories daily remind us of jobs not being done properly.

What we may not recognise is that from the staff point of view, they have become the filler in a club sandwich. Along with their own pressures within and without the wards, the tenuous nature of employment in the NHS and the godlike status of this mythical sacred cow, their own vulnerability is rarely brought into question. Why? they are humans too. With Governments, patients, senior colleagues, and public expectation and the media, they do well to survive and perform as well as they do, professional or otherwise.

Surgical interventions like hip replacements, appendectomies, hernias and the like are one thing for doctors and nurses, even relatives. They are fairly predictable and require relatively brief stays in hospital. Staff can feel that it is a case of "a good job done" when people leave the wards, but are often more challenged when a mysterious and apparently incurable situation confronts them on a daily basis. People who have to visit their loved ones over many weeks, even months, often develop a kind of compassion fatigue as the weeks go by. I have seen very faithful families at the bedside day after day. I have also seen many looking more and more tired as the weeks go on. I regularly saw mothers under particular stress with a sick child knowing that other children are at home receiving care from grandparents or partners who have to get time off work. The strain tells. It can be like siege conditions while it lasts, particularly parental overnight stays in the paediatric wards. You can understand perfectly well why any relationships might get strained when children are separated from their parents and one sibling is given much more attention than others.

Further changes can develop in relationships when expectations of length of hospital stay change. The expected time span for support can change the way in people view their commitment to visit. The open-ended nature of some cancer treatments is a case in point. For some families, life can actually revolve around a relative's condition and the visit to the hospital becomes as much of the week as a trip to the supermarket. For the cancer patient chemotherapy and blood transfusions may happen regularly, so that a particular week may be given over to post treatment recovery. Helpfully many units are Day Case and it is like just like going to the hairdresser. You go, have the necessary treatment and leave. Those with kidney disease and require dialysis cannot expect to live life like others. They are governed by the 'clock' of their treatment. Casual friends often visit with enthusiasm at the beginning but their visits fall off once they realise that this may be an indefinite process. This is hard for the patient. Often they cannot voice it. They may have to carry their sadness inside.

A particular problem for visitors is the actual length of a stay when visiting. I see this all the time, and the experience is affirmed by many patients. When a person has taken the trouble to visit and found a parking space and paid for it, or taken two buses to get to hospital, they want to give a 'value for money' visit. Many visitors will run out of conversation after fifteen minutes and many patients just get tired out when they overstay their time. I have often heard a weariness coming from patients who are caught between gratitude for someone coming, and frustration that they just won't leave! Both health professionals and pastoral workers need to recognise that if a person is not well, it tires them to keep up a conversation. Even friends and relations will find there are growth points to face in the business of visiting with sensitivity. Keeping visits short and sweet may also keep relationships harmonious and health promoting rather than energy sapping!

CARE OF CARERS?

For many reasons 'compassion fatigue' is common. We cannot judge anyone for this. We are only human. It is particularly acute for the principal carers of disabled people and those with special needs or mental health problems. It may be easier said than done, but carers should need to take care of *themselves* as well as caring for their sick friend or relative. It does nobody any good to wear themselves into the ground and get seriously depleted. Hospital wards are full of people who are carers themselves and anxious to get better in order to care for another. I think sometimes that it is the weight of caring that has been partly responsible for putting there in the first place. I wonder often whether this pressure is a barrier to recovery

It is sometimes very appropriate to do "shifts" in long term visiting. The family decides at the beginning of the week which person should go on which day. This seems profoundly sensible. This 'rota' system refreshes people and gives them renewed energy and even new things to talk about to the patient, and it also safeguards relationships.

To understand some of these things is necessary to anyone seeking to draw alongside the sick, whether professionally or in a more family or pastoral capacity. Chaplaincy in hospital concerns itself with spiritual care, but that can be expressed in very ordinary conversations and even meaningful silences. The Holistic and Spiritual Care Policy that drives our own work states the case: " Spiritual care addresses the basic human need for a sense of hope, purpose and meaning in the midst of the anxiety often related to the experience of hospitalisation"(22) What lies beneath the presenting medical problem, is the person who needs support.

The hospital's space for healing is only on loan. Most people do not stay forever in their wards. But for many the environment does take a bit of getting used to, and it bring a largely hidden aspect of life, being ill, not in control and out of the swim, painfully into the present. Those close to patients are involved in their loved one's adjustment. Anyone visiting may find themselves meeting people struggling with the whole business.

9

THE NEED FOR PERSONAL CONTROL IN LIFE

Illness may be found to be stealing your world as well. Unless people have been disabled from birth or brought up in an extremely controlling family atmosphere, they will have gained some independence as individuals as they grow up. This will be shown by getting a job or going on to further education, finding a partner or moving away from home. As life progresses people gather the people and things around them that suit their tastes, personalities and interests. Freedom of choice may rule OK in many areas of the outside world but not always in the ward!

One shock that coming into hospital brings is the lack of control over one's environment. In hospital you cannot eat just when you want to. Your diet may be governed by investigative tests, operations, observations, and of course, set meal times. To begin with there may be a novelty factor in this, but after a while the inevitable institutionalisation can become burdensome, even oppressive. Depending on peoples' tolerance this experience can bring out considerable anger or the onset of reactive depression.

The patient experiences that the space they possess on the ward, with bed, locker and table is only theirs for a limited period. Before them it 'belonged' to someone else. This space is also an open door to whatever healthcare professional may choose to come along. In reality it is not really their 'special' space at all. Nowhere is, except the bathroom or toilet, and only then for a short while. This erosion of privacy can leave people vulnerable or resentful. Certainly it may give someone the sense that their own home is very nice indeed. In the course of a year I hear the phrase "There's no place like home" repeated several hundred times. People do really get to love their homes more than ever when separated from them in hospital. Of course there is a minority of people who live entirely alone, and for whom hospital presents a social opportunity unknown in their ordinary lives. As human beings we need a measure of control in our lives though. When it is taken away, we might feel angry or vulnerable.

SICKNESS IS A THIEF

The fact is that illness can not only steal a person's physical and emotional wellbeing, but also their everyday normality. The patient's world literally shrinks. Because we will not be aware of this we mostly see it as the downside of having treatment. Many give up as a silent protest against having little control over their life. What I see among many elderly people, in particular, is often a gradual withdrawal from the world around them because they cannot come to terms with their environment. This withdrawal can express itself as a resigned switching off from the institutionalism, lack of privacy and limited choice in activity. I have often spent time with an elderly person who seems to have gone on 'standby' mode, yet found at the end of a two way conversation for ten minutes, that person has 'come back' and once more taken an interest in the world. The presence of a chaplaincy service and volunteer visitors is vital in hospitals for this kind of restorative intervention. Staff can sometimes be too caught up in necessary tasks to observe this waning of attentiveness in individuals.

Spiritual care is essential to address the consequences of coming into hospital. Just by listening to a person's story, hearing a little about what they like or don't like 'normalises' them. They feel like people again. Spiritual care delivers a slice of 'normality' to those suffering as a result of illness, accident or elective operation because it is open ended, less concerned with the physical 'nuts and bolts' and addresses the essence of a person. What enlivens them and makes them tick. It puts them on the map. It can stay with the pain of those struggling with an unwelcome physical condition in an alien environment. To value the whole 'person in the patient' with their anxieties, disorientation and changed circumstances requires empathy and time. To recognise this alongside the medical and surgical attention, is to truly enhance the patient experience, and help to 'keep them together' during this time. It can give them a little

40

bit of control back, because they are listened to. To repeat the catch phrase it is *value added*.

BUT THE *RIGHT* PLACE TOO

And now the good news... yes, there is most definitely an up side in being in hospital.. The flow of this book up till now may appear rather negative towards the hospital experience. The truth is that when a person is ill, they are in the right place when they are admitted. That was certainly my experience when I had acute pneumonia. I felt like death. I was worried. My temperature was over 104 for four days. The ambulance taking me into the unknown had the effect of making me feel safe on that occasion. I know many relatives who breathe a collective sigh of relief when their loved one is safely in a hospital bed. The care and the expertise is present there to assess and diagnose and successfully treat them. Second opinions are also on hand in hospitals. It is a place of reassuring attention for the unwell and generally a comfort for the anxious and frightened. For those who have been waiting a long time for an operation, the primary objective has been to get a bed. Now they have achieved their goal, there is a sense that the rest will follow.

Hospitals are places where people expect to come, get treated and go home as soon as possible. They are not generally conceived of as long stay environments, though in fact we know they can be. The context of hospitals is that of hope. This hope that people bring to it connects with the hope that doctors, nurses and therapists also bring to the working environment. This synergy generated by patient and staff encourages expectation, and although this cannot always be realised, nonetheless it prevails as the predominant ethos of this setting.

Health is a delicate matter. I have already established that. However, the health of one person inevitably touches the lives of other people. Some people have indefinable health problems for years such as the post viral syndrome termed ME. Even specialists have been divided in their opinion of this post viral fatigue syndrome. Eventually there emerged a test that clearly identified this alien in the bloodstream and the physical and psychosocial changes it brings. Perhaps bewildered by

41

the symptoms and guided by the lack of agreement among the medical profession, partners of the afflicted and senior work colleagues might have been disparaging to them in the early days. This of course heaped further pressures on the sick people and stress further debilitated them. It is quite lonely and hurtful not to be believed by others.

Being admitted to hospital under these conditions gives something back to people who are being misunderstood. Becoming treated means they have been believed. They are not seen as crying wolf, which is a fear many have. It is as if a seal of approval is granted in the recognition of an actual illness or condition. Even a diagnosis based on exhaustive tests can give back some of the eroded self-esteem to a person who is undermined by the doubts in others. Hospital puts brackets round that person and tells them, "it is all right for you to be incapacitated, there really is something wrong with you." That can bring great relief to people and in also to employers and family. These are ways in which illness and hospitalisation does not steal a person's self-worth, but confers some sense of vindication for them.

10

THE TRAUMA OF BECOMING A PATIENT

"This is ME you know!" How often might we want to stand up and shout this in a hospital ward, when our feelings convey that something important in *us* is being eroded by this experience.

Is a patient a person? Ten years ago we employed a number of Filipino nurses as home grown nursing stocks were getting low. I was asked to be a part of the induction. In order to do my homework I asked around. How do we do it here differently? One overseas health care worker commented to me that in the Philippines "We treat the person, but here in the U.K. you treat the condition." Therein is an important difference in perception. Today increasingly, public health care has come to resemble a "biological garage". The 'patient experience' of this process naturally concentrates on the focused attention given by the medical staff to speedy and efficient diagnosis and treatment. Nonetheless it is easy to lose sight in this desire to treat people with speed of the *person in the patient*. The health care received whilst you are a 'body in transit' is only part of the human need at that point. The best health care is that which will recognise and treat the whole person, mind, body, soul and spirit. I repeat that well- being is much more than being well. I may be overstating the case but many of us who have witnessed exemplary moments of hospital care, will still have had some idea of the picture I am describing here. Robin Youngson makes the point in relation to the differing approaches of healthcare; "There is a world of difference between open-hearted compassion with non-attachment and the western model of clinical detachment, which leaves patients feeling so abandoned."(23)

John Taylor puts it very well as he observed back in the 1970s, "Now it is perfectly true that when the surgeon is actually bent over my inert body I do not want his concentration distracted by any feelings of dislike or admiration. But if on approaching my bed a few days later, he refers to me as "the gall bladder", I feel alienated. I am glad to be his object, his problem, on the operating table – but I am not simply ' a problem', or 'an object once I come round."(24)

When several years of study and training for doctors and nursing staff have concentrated around on text books, diagrams, lectures 'about' conditions, pathologies and the dissection of dead bodies, it is not surprising that junior doctors particularly, for all their vocational enthusiasm, might baulk at the actual patient who is living, dynamic and sometimes a bit truculent. Emotional intelligence is vital when dealing with vulnerable people. This is perhaps an unfair comment on the dedication of most doctors and nurses, but observation over several years has led to the view that sometimes the personal is lost in the clinical. The focus in modern healthcare has to be on the person who has the disease and not solely on the disease or condition itself, however interesting. That person needs to be recognised in their social and emotional context which includes their family and community and even their day job. Canon Peter Speck, a chaplain for 30 years commented during his address in a celebration of Healthcare Chaplaincy at Manchester Cathedral recently that very early in his career, "a lady in a side room seen by a dozen people on the morning she was admitted, all of whom examined parts of her. I was the end of the line. She was reading a magazine. She didn't look up as I introduced myself but threw back the bedclothes and said "which bit do you want?" to which I replied "I want all of you" and thankfully she laughed.

The clinical and sometimes rather impersonal approach to people and their health problems is often referred to as 'the medical model' of medicine, as opposed to the pastoral and holistic model. Healthcare needs a marriage of both. The following extract from an 80 year old patient's letter illustrates this further. "I felt like a packet of biscuits being hurled from one place to another . . . I never thought that I would one day be known simply as a patient number."

I once went onto a respiratory Ward and heard an alarming indictment of patient care from one particular person. I met a young man in his thirties who confided that every morning he went into the ward toilets on a daily basis and cried. His comment to me was "they just don't seem to realise that we have feelings." I do not doubt the sincerity of that man's experience at all, but I doubt whether he was entirely accurate in his perception of his treatment, being in a highly emotional and fragmented state. Although I have heard the same story on many occasions, I think the real issue is often about the understaffing of wards, and the resulting haste and stress that is visibly present. If there are too many patients to attend to, too many jobs to do, when another patient calls out, a dread often arises in nurses that they will forget the last thing they had to do. Also, I do believe that when it comes to the genuine feelings of patients needing attention many of the nursing staff do not want to get sucked into what they imagine will be a very draining and time absorbing distraction from the 'tyranny of the urgent' under which they have to operate. It is not deliberate ill-will that denied this man a hearing or human empathy, but the system; the institutional malaise. It may be observed on occasions that the nursing station or rest room is literally serving as a place of retreat for staff who are understandably burdened by constant need. Some calls for assistance, bells pressed and 'vexatious complainants' will from time to time be avoided by the use of selective deafness. However the question may need to be asked, when does avoidance border on neglect?

A colleague passed on an experience that highlights the fact that to recognise people as fellow human beings is so important within the institution. On arriving at the hospital one morning in late summer, he told me that he encountered a gentleman of later middle age who was seated in the foyer outside the chaplaincy office. They made introductions, during which the man explained that he was semi-retired clergyman who still volunteered some time in chaplaincy at a nearby hospital. As the conversation developed my colleague referred to the Trust's recently adopted Holistic and Spiritual Healthcare Policy. Picking up on the term "holistic" this man described his experiences of healthcare from General Practitioners to Hospital Consultants over the last six months.

BEING HEARD

Because of a number of conditions, he had consultations with

45

over twenty clinicians, but the most significant visit for him was with one who talked, questioned and actively listened, seeking to know something of his story, lifestyle and their effects upon his physical and emotional health. And then the crunch: the doctor looked at him and said "Right, let's take a look at it." The man then said to my colleague, "In that moment I was healed. I felt better right away."

Seemingly no one else had wanted to examine his foot, nor had they shown interest in anything other than specific symptoms. This other doctor's approach was focused and concentrated but above all holistic. The man wasn't a "numb foot" he was a *person*.

11

THE TRAUMA OF LOSING LIFE'S LANDMARKS

Disorientation is a common experience on the wards. Amidst all the signs, instructions and the guides who accompany people to elusive destinations, people do find most hospitals maze-like. It can be most disorientating. Sometimes hospitals are places more akin to a foreign land, than health restoring, people friendly places of healing. The socially appropriate and connecting landmarks can be surprisingly absent sometimes.

Smells, instrumentation, shared sleeping accommodation and the constant monitoring by health professionals make a hospital, far from home as it is, a place of threat as well as one of treatment and healing. Many people pine for home, particularly those with a poor understanding of why they are in hospital in the first place. To suddenly encounter poor health is bad enough, but when hospitals feel like a foreign land where the language and customs are far from familiar to the new arrival, it is trauma.

Many of us have been fortunate enough to have been abroad for our holidays or on business trips. Even in these days of social and cultural similarities we will immediately recognise that there are many differences around us when we emerge from the airport, station or port. We notice that the signs and advertisements are different, in language and in style. The cars will probably drive on a different side of the road. The further we probe into the country the more the differences emerge and they will have an impact on us. Different sounds, smells and atmospheres all conjure up a picture of 'somewhere else, not home'. Some of this will surprise us pleasantly, like fine weather, tempting food smells and delicious fragrances from herbs and flowers. Others will confuse and disorientate us, like the language, road signs and protocols involved in crossing the road or queuing at a shop. A foreign land, we shall probably find, is a place that we need to get used to. We may not immediately feel settled and at home with everything. Even doing basic activities like shopping or asking directions to where we want to go can get confusing or even threatening abroad. We can often feel small, like being children again. Vulnerability, a sense of alienation or even distress may accompany our first days in another country.

A similar experience may meet those who are admitted to hospital. To many a hospital is just like a foreign land. Immediately a person can recognise that a hospital is both institutional and a complicated environment to negotiate. There will be countless signs telling us which way to go, using slightly technical language like "Cardiorespiratory Outpatients" and "Day-Case Unit" or "GUM". As often as not, the place that people need to find is not one of the signs that is displayed. They may need to ask someone. Feeling a bit small and lost in such a large institution is actually quite normal. I experience it myself when visiting other hospitals. Inside these buildings it is easy to find oneself bewildered by the many directions displayed. If a hospital re-sites an Outpatients Department or Pathology where bloods are taken, for instance, it can totally confuse people who are familiar with the old layout until they get used to the new arrangements.

HOSPITALS INC.

The institutional side of a hospital building will make itself evident very soon. Even a Shopping Centre is easier to find your way around. Perhaps a hospital compares with a large busy airport upon first arrival. "It's just like a departure lounge at an airport" were the exact words countless visitors used when describing the entrance of our newly built hospital. It gives a much more 'commercial' ambience than that of the quiet hotel atmosphere of many hospices for instance. There are very definite signals given by this design. To begin, as I have mentioned before, it is not like home. It is more like an alien environment, unless you are a frequent flier! As I have said disorientation is a common feeling at first. I spend minutes every week redirecting lost patients and families, clutching their appointment letters and looking bewildered, to the Department they need. It is not always easy to stop purposeful looking people in uniform striding in a focused manner down a hospital corridor. Often the feeling of "I ought to know" comes into one's head and seals our lips unnecessarily. The truth is, that most health care workers are only too happy to point you in the right direction, in the same way as the average person in a foreign city will help you find your destination. It takes courage though, to ask. Entering hospital usually does not fill us with courage!

The bustling Accident and Emergency Department in a hospital for instance may also be likened to a foreign port, airport or station. When a person is admitted to this department, it may feel like nothing they have experienced before. When I was admitted to St.Bartholomew's Hospital in London in 1977, it was from an ambulance journey which was rather scary. I spent a lot of time in a bay behind curtains, hearing sounds but wondering what was going on and what was going to happen to me next. In many ways I was 'in their hands'. Of course many people will be only too glad to receive medical attention. They will feel that despite the strangeness, they are in the right place. Some people will have a deep seated fear of hospitals, or 'white coat syndrome.' We are all different. After an hour or two in a cubicle, I personally experienced increased feelings of anxiety. There for a time my questioning inevitably increased. In this situation for most people the chorus of uncertainties is likely to echo in their heads; "What is happening?" "Will I be kept in?" "What is wrong with me?"

Thankfully these departments in which new patients are seen have improved so much in past years over the speed with which people are seen and sent to the next destination, whether home or a ward or the operating theatre. The Government has until recently stipulated a four hour "turnaround" time. People were admitted, triaged (assessed for level of seriousness), X-rayed (if necessary) and see a clinician before assessment as to what treatment should follow. Under the phenomenon known as 'winter bed pressures' sometimes the wait can be much longer and even corridors may become temporary wards. Most of us have probably experienced that energy sapping experience in the Accident and Emergency waiting room staring at the LED display announcing the daunting number of minutes that the department estimates it will be before you are seen. All the while strange events may be going on around you, as people come off the streets with bloody injuries or noisy relatives; not the best surroundings at the best of times. Throughout the buildings you get a sense of the well-run, highly organised yet very busy day to day functioning of an institution that has a job to do. The feeling of the institutional is much more marked here than in say, a hospice, which is so much smaller and hotel-like.

FROM PRIVATE TO SHARED

Once a person has got beyond the stage of taking in the new experience of being in hospital, there is the experience of ward itself. Many people of course, are admitted routinely onto a ward, particularly if the time has come for an elective operation. Nonetheless there is a world of difference between a hospital ward and everyday life. New hospitals usually have four or five bedded wards that are fresh and modern, and give off messages about efficiency, good hygiene and professionalism. There are still many Victorian buildings that have been given countless makeovers that will never disguise their antique roots. The older ones may well still have "Nightingale Wards" with upwards of 25 beds in them, with perhaps a couple of side wards off the main one. The logic of this probably goes back to the Crimean War and the influence of Florence Nightingale in the military field hospitals. It is all about organisation and efficiency. It is easier in these wards though for the nursing station to keep an eye on proceedings, but they can be quite daunting to be admitted onto. There have been wards in my own Trust where there were 30 beds, if you count the main ward and side wards. Thankfully the new building, opened in 2010, has done away with this. These large wards become noisy at night because patients are admitted overnight which is disturbing for light sleepers, and the occasionally noisy patient usually succeeds in keeping others awake.

It doesn't take much to imagine the feelings of anxiety and vulnerability that may arise in these circumstances. Add to it the fact of illness when a person 'just doesn't want to know.' If you consider the strangeness of the ward environment there is a big adjustment to be made for the new patient. Even in a small ward you are "sharing" your bedroom with three or four others! Looking out on a number of other patients suffering various degrees of sickness may be demoralising to a new patient. The geography of the bed is also alien to the newcomer. Other patients may have drips, catheter bags and post operational lines running from their necks; particularly unnerving to the new arrival. There may be drains to draw off fluids from surgical procedures. To see all this upon admission can be a culture shock. The total impact of all these changes is the realisation that this is an alien experience; a far cry from the domesticity that they will have left to come into hospital.

An illustration of the kind of alienation felt by some patients became very clear to me one day I entered a ward. It came from a lady I had already visited for over six months. She described an episode that was sadly repeated many times during her stay and she kindly wrote it down for me to record.

"The last two evenings have been a nightmare. The woman in bed 6 has dementia. She calls out all night in a loud voice and instead of feeling compassion for her I resent her because for two nights the only thing I know as home, "my corner" or my space has been invaded once more and I know it is going to mean sleep deprivation for me, and I am worrying for my own sanity." It isn't hard to feel the mounting stress in that lady's experience.

The change in status

The change from ordinary life in entering hospital can mirror that from being an adult to becoming a child again. Describing one patient's experience in the United States, coming from a farming background to a highly technological place like a hospital, Henri Nouwen has written: "It must have been like coming to another planet where the people dress, behave, talk and act in a frightfully strange way. The white nurses, with their efficient way of washing, feeding and dressing patients; the doctors with their charts, making notes and giving orders in an utterly strange language; the many unidentifiable machines with bottles and tubes; and all the strange smells, noises and foods must have made Mr Harrison feel like a little child who has lost his way in a fearful forest." (25) When you look at what happens to a person when they come into hospital, you are reminded of a sequence of events that gradually strips the autonomy from a person. The same pattern occurs irrespective of who the person is, whether a bank manager, a mum with young children, a student, a homeless person or someone in the manufacturing industry or building trade. They come into the institution from the outside world where they have some measure of control in their lives in to enter a state of dependency. Their clothes have to be exchanged from recognisably personal every day wear to nightclothes. Like a child they go to bed, they are told (very nicely) what they must do and when they must do it, and then the ordinary freedoms of life disappear.

The next stage may feel like a regression into childhood. Personal autonomy and some sense of independence is slowly eroded. Clinicians will come and see them, some with great empathy and helpfulness, and clarity, explaining simply what will happen. Others might arrive at the bedside exhibiting a slightly more remote bearing and using inaccessible medical language which leaves a person feeling more alienated, isolated and vulnerable. There are times when the patient starts to ask questions or make requests that they can be made to feel sometimes like naughty children. Thankfully this is not the norm. I realise these descriptions may not always be seen as the ones that every patient will identify with, but from my experience many certainly will. I am not trying to blame anyone particular for what is characteristic of most institutions, but sometimes it is the price we pay for a National Health Service that treats countless people under pressured conditions. Of course there needs to be efficient management systems to deal with the intense human need represented, but the processes of admission such as the ones described may also run the risk of demeaning people and causing them to feel they are in a state of exile, where there is little privacy

"Psychologically and spiritually" defines Marcus Borg, "exile is a condition of alienation, a sense of being cut off from a centre of meaning and energy"(26) This may explain why perhaps a kind of lethargy can fall upon particularly vulnerable patients, especially those for whom the trauma of being hospitalised is felt most deeply. Oddly enough, those who are most active and perhaps self- sufficient in the outside world may be most affected. It is like the clipping of their wings, and where impotence is not a usual experience and they may find that they have no answer to that. Our support as chaplains or visitors may be simply that of recognising the inwardness of this difficult condition and enable these people to put words to it.

HOME-LESS

One of the most common phrases I hear from the patients is that "there is no place like home." Some even sing the familiar old song to me to prove their point. This is a revelation to ordinary people who suddenly find themselves diminished by this hospital experience, an environment that is simply very different from anything else. This sense of "home" is the preserve of most people. We should not underestimate what comfort it brings. It helps to define us as people. Its value is so often heightened by being away from it. At home you are surrounded by the familiar. In hospital you are not. At home choices can be made; what and when to eat, what to drink, what to do and when to go to the toilet or bathe. Hospitals are by necessity more regimented and cannot compete with most homes for user friendliness. Away from home people can experience "homesickness". As I mentioned before, home defines who you are, and when home seems a very long way off, you can experience feelings of loss and vulnerability which in metaphysical terms might be described as a 'sickness of the heart'.

Homesickness is not a term used much today. The experience of it is. During the last century those evacuated during the Second World War would have been familiar with the experience, as well as those in the Armed Forces overseas. It can be acute with those those have been sent away to boarding school at a tender age or possibly those who find themselves in prison (unconscious connection?) or leaving home for the first time as a young adult. Separation anxiety is not only for the young. With separation can come a pining for the home, the familiar and that place of belonging that helps us to recognise who we are and our place on the map.

Many who are elderly and confused can begin to 'fragment' emotionally when they are away from their familiar surroundings, whether be it their own home or a residential home. This is particularly difficult when admission to hospital happens hurriedly. When we visit patients in hospital, as people who can offer pastoral support, we need to be aware of this aspect of loss that affects many patients. They will not be fully settled just because they are in a place that can offer them treatment and hope, and we need to understand that to support them better.

It is evident when you see patients in their beds how the nature of their stay is transitional and not permanent. However their new environment is definitely not home for them. For one thing they can only take a few personal items with them. If they are not rushed in then they can pack a small bag or case, but if a General Practitioner admits them from their surgery or a person collapses in a Shopping Centre then it might be up to relatives to bring in the necessary toiletries and personal effects. As often or not it takes several attempts to get that right! If someone's admission is a blue light job then the chances are that feelings of disorientation might be even greater because of the adrenalin charge of such events, unless of course the person is unconscious. This and other surprise elements can induce panic. If a person is confused in any way, a sense of "where am I?" prevails. Further to this, without some of their own personal items they will probably be given a hospital marked nightgown which further erodes a sense of personal identity. There is a real sense of wellbeing that comes from just having "one's own stuff" there, little though it may be it helps to define us and provide a small part of home.

REMINISCENCE; RESTORING LANDMARKS

To remember means literally to re-member; to put oneself together again. This is a vital therapy when losing one's bearings in hospital. One particular occupational therapist discovered the value of getting patients to talk about their past. For years she ran reminiscence groups, so that as many people who were not bedbound would gather in a circle and various artifacts from years ago such as washing and cooking products were passed round. People would tell their tales of how it was for them in their particular day. They were able to handle bars of carbolic, medicines, cleaning products and magazines of the

1950's. This was a good example of spiritual care because it allowed people, exiled, say from the familiar to experience things that were meaningful to them in terms of their lives. A Reminiscence Room was opened at the back of one ward. It was typical of the front room in around 1949, and some of these groups took place there. It was opened by the Mayor of Wakefield and we celebrated Her Majesty the Queen's Golden Jubilee in it with tea and cake! Sadly the room fell into disuse as the occupational therapist was appointed to a new role and pressures on the space grew. However it later became a day room, rather cluttered and pulled back into the institution. A little bit of welcome nostalgia has now gone.

I also remember, on other rehabilitation wards holding little Songs of Praise at Christmas, Easter and Harvest time with an accompanist, again as a familiar feature for many elderly people. So often they would be wheeled into the largest space in the ward area saying "Oh, I can't sing", but within a few moments of a favourite hymn striking up they were singing heartily. Probably these occasions were more of a 'normalising' feature than anything seriously religious, but for many it brought their pasts into the present, along with an awareness of their own special identity. I believe all these things constituted a holistic and spiritual care for elderly and disorientated patients. The cost to provide them was negligible, but the time to run them had to end when rehabilitation was all moved, and folk went into wards with no piano.

12

THE TRAUMA OF PATIENT POWER EROSION

In our desire to make patients feel at home and cared for, a prime error staff may fall into is that of taking away their wishes, even at the simplest level. Many elderly people who have referred to lifelong neighbours as '*Mrs Jones*' or '*Mr Tompkins*' may be quite upset at enforced intimacies. However good staff may feel about addressing the new patient as "Hello Doris", perhaps Doris may feel stripped naked as a result of this well intentioned address. They should be asked. Although I have witnessed a shift in the name plates over beds from intimate to more formal, it might preserve people's dignity to tell them upon admission, "We will address you as Miss Smith, until you tell us otherwise." The choice and the dignity will then rest with the patient.

Another prime example of the sense of potential powerlessness that can creep into the experience of the individual in hospital is where possessions "walk". Money, clothes, glasses and hearing aids and dentures can go missing. It is not always the result of foul play. Some items get scooped up in bed linen, while others disappear during a transition from one ward to another. I have never known of a huge cache of these things in hospital, but there must be a haul of them somewhere like an elephants graveyard!

To illustrate this, an apocryphal tale was told which described how a new nurse was once very keen to show her nursing superiors that she was keen and responsible. This was her first ward. A senior staff member picked up on her willingness and assigned her to get the dentures cleaned on the ward while the patients were asleep. She set about this task with great enthusiasm and gusto, placing them all on a tray and taking them along to where she could clean them. She performed the cleaning with precision and vigour. Believing this to be a good job done, and being ready to return them to their slumbering owners' lockers she suddenly came to the awful realisation that in her enthusiasm to collect them she had kept no record of whom they individually belonged to! She sheepishly reported this back to her senior staff member who had to redeem the situation, much to the amusement of her other colleagues. Apocryphal or not, these things happen. Somehow I cannot think that her vulnerable patients would have all seen the funny side of the folly of her youthful enthusiasm. With dentures, one size certainly doesn't fit all!

I also remember a time when a particular penny dropped with an elderly lady I had seen for a few weeks. She noticed that something seemed amiss. She was the sort of person who did not want to put anyone to any trouble. She just mentioned in passing that she had been transferred from one ward to another, but she was sure she had her glasses when she was in the other ward. Since then they had gone missing. I checked on her previous ward and after searching in the places they might have been the staff drew a blank. I told her and she seemed baffled but accepted the matter. It was when she asked me particular questions about the flowers on the table and which nurse had just passed by I realised she was nearly blind. Her glasses helped give her some control in her situation. Losing them disabled her. I further discovered that she did have another pair at a residential home where she lived. I happened to know the place, having visited it before, so shortly after, tying it in with a bereavement visit nearby I dropped in to claim her glasses. The difference to her was astonishing. She brightened up in wonder as for the first time she could actually see her surroundings. For her it was better than winning the lottery, but what a simple provision. I just wish I had seen it earlier. The tragedy was that nobody else had! Spiritual care, as we shall look at later, is often about simple, practical things. These too can lift the spirits.

A DROP OF HUMANITY

The ward routine, for all the most understandable reasons is not like home either. It can leave us feeling like pawns in a larger system. Hospitals have to be institutional. Meals arrive at certain times. Tea or coffee is served between these points. The library trolley, sweet trolley and paper trolley will all appear during the morning. Then there is visiting time. In between all these are trips to the bathroom and toilet, often nursing support. Then there will be procedures, tests and scans, often accessed by chair taken by a porter. Apart from the delays, waits and cancellations there is a sense of clockwork running through hospital life, where the individual gradually surrenders their own sense of autonomy, and even worse their sense of self. In terms of spiritual healthcare, we need to recognise the effect the institutional side of things has on the individual.

Such is a hospital. It is a place that is not like home. It is actually more like a foreign land. With good care and observation, the environment can certainly be improved upon. Being aware of and acknowledging these issues, should be part of the basic understanding of all healthcare workers, and it would certainly help those in the beds who cannot find their own words for the experience. When we visit patients with the intention of supporting them, we may not be prepared for what they may require from us. Self- awareness and empathy is the key. As long as we can remain in touch with our own humanity we will do what is necessary. A chaplain describes an episode that illustrates the gift of touching another's situation with sensitivity. A woman the chaplain was visiting in a surgical ward would endure serious pain spasms for a few seconds. The conversation would halt until she was ready to continue. Then suddenly the patient grabbed the chaplain's hand which had been carefully placed so that it could be held if so wished, closed her eyes and went rigid. Chaplain and patient sat in shared silence. When she was ready to speak all she said was "Thank you for not walking away when I was in pain." It is this level of knowing that can so bridge the gap between a difficult experience, and one where a sense of "at home-ness" can prevail. The quality of our engagement matters. It is, in the end something that is more to do with interpersonal relationships than technique. Through developing compassionate awareness by engaging as fellow human beings with our patients we can certainly reinforce a realistically caring environment.

13

THE TRAUMA OF FEELING FRAGILE

Feeling uncomfortable in the healthcare setting is not unusual. Many people are quite private about their bodies, and what affects them. Modesty and dignity though are what hospitals normally strive for. The vision of only single sex wards is slowly becoming a reality, but from time to time we can be caught out. Admissions wards are particularly difficult to segregate because of course, no one can know just who is going to be given a bed and where it will be at any point in the day or night.

A patient from a different culture may well find the challenges to modesty quite difficult even offensive. Muslim patients will expect high standards of respect and same-sex medical attention as well as ward privacy. As I have mentioned the days of mixed wards are thankfully coming to an end. Cultural sensitivity, whilst enshrined in NHS Policy can easily break down through the sheer pressure of necessity. Having alluded to this fact in the previous chapter it is obvious that at home people do not have to share their bedrooms with strangers. Unless you are assigned to a single room for some reason, this is still quite normal in hospital. Many find the experience very disconcerting and sometimes frightening and it requires a big adjustment to accept this aspect of the hospital experience.

One obvious example of institutional immodesty is right there in front of us and may surprise the observant newly admitted patient or an outpatient on route to a procedure. Many will have seen those surgical gowns that open at the back, in which some patients have to walk to surgery, unaware that their modesty is being compromised from the gaping void behind where there are no tie strings. This, of course gives a whole new meaning to the term 'ICU' which sounds just like *"I see you"*- hardly what our privacy and dignity protocols require! We may see the funny side of this; vulnerable patients generally don't.

Apart from the unfamiliar nature of the sleeping quarters and the strange instrumentation that routinely adorn the wards, the patient may also be aware of a new experience; they have no front door to their new 'home'. Family and visitors may take for granted this new aspect of their loved ones' environment, but the ready access that anyone can have to their bedside may cause some patients an element of surprise, even shock. Respect, which is close to having value (see Spiritual Needs List: Chapter 5) is actually a spiritual need. It speaks about the value of a person. We breach this at our peril as a caring organisation, and at the cost of adding insult to injury to the patient. When any health professional approaches a patient in their bed it is unusual for them to ask permission to enter their bedside area. This could be seen as actually a breach of respect, but one that is unlikely to cut much ice with those who need to see the patient urgently. After all, that is why the doctor is in there in the first place, and that is why the patient is available in bed.

All approaches and interventions are considered to be fair game for the health professionals, doctor, nurse, phlebotomist, physiotherapist, chaplain or whoever. However, from the patient's point of view, their rights are automatically breached once people to go through their 'front door' unannounced. This assumption that the patient is somehow the hospital's property calls into question this issue of respect. It also impinges on the matter of privacy. I was brought to book once by an elderly man who asked "And who are you?" I showed him my clerical collar and ID explaining I was a chaplain making a routine visit to the ward. He was not impressed and told me in no uncertain terms that I should have announced myself and my purpose clearly before expecting to carry on a conversation. I remembered this for a while, but I have to admit that I regularly forgot the niceties. Perhaps a case of my being over familiar with the job!

I have spoken about the issue of mixed wards that are being phased out. Trusts are fined when they operate them, which is a powerful incentive these days. As a now endangered species they and assessment wards are likely to have both men and women in close proximity. When an ill person comes into hospital and has to change into nightclothes and get into bed, often the last thing that they require for their peace of mind when the curtains are drawn back is a member of the opposite sex across the room from them. It happens. The other thing about admissions wards is that they are holding wards. They are not usually the patient's final destination. As people are admitted any time of day or night, they are difficult places to get rest. There is also the issue of people's vulnerability. The last thing anyone wants when feeling ill is disturbance. Some patients can be very disruptive for many reasons, alcohol being a principal one, and it is not uncommon for Hospital Security to have to come onto admissions wards to "sort out" some rumpus or other. This is traumatic for the anxious and unwell person as well as nursing staff.

RESPECT FOR CULTURAL AND RELIGIOUS NEED

The questions of modesty and privacy are naturally felt keenly by many patients in hospital. I believe hospitals need to continually remind themselves of this as they seek to do everything that might make their patients comfortable. Thank goodness for the curtains around the bed, though it is often pretty clear what is going on behind them when they are closed, especially when a commode has just been brought in. These issues have been highlighted in order to respond to the presence on the wards of patients from other cultures for which privacy is paramount. Quality care is about getting details like this right. A certain level of privacy and modesty is undoubtedly the prerogative of the patient.

The Muslim chaplains have been much used in the Trust I worked for. Not only do they address the issues of modesty, they often find themselves addressing the issue of "how can I be a good Muslim in hospital?" This means ensuring the food for Muslim patients is *halal*; that particular medications were free from pig products and advising on the degree to which daily prayers can be accommodated in hospital. As Moulana Ilyas Dalal says " I receive calls from patients who are concerned about taking Enoxaprin (Clexane/Lovenox) because it is derived from pork. I tell patients that they need to take it. Even though it is forbidden to eat pork, taking this medicine is not a problem because Islamic Law is more flexible in these types of situations than we may think." (27)

Further issues that create a feeling of vulnerability for Muslim families are the protocols surrounding birth, death and burial. Being reassured that particular religious needs are being addressed in the right way leads more of a feeling of being 'at home' in the hospital setting, thus promoting dignity and respect and allaying anxiety. The chaplaincy, which is interdenominational and multi-faith developed a 'Faiths and Practice' laminated sheet in 1998 for the wards, to help with protocols with those of different cultures and religions. This sheet deals with such matters as diet, festivals, ablutions, language, modesty and protocols around death. Many staff have told us that they have been help by this simple tool when they have felt uncomfortable, not quite knowing how to proceed in some situations.

ALL SORTS AND CONDITIONS ...

Hospitals of course will admit anyone in need of immediate and acute clinical care. The Trust will usually have an Equality and Diversity Policy in place which basically means we try not to adopt a prejudicial attitude towards certain people. However, among those patients admitted are those we might term as being "vulnerable persons." Now as we know, *all* patients are vulnerable, not just specially selected and identified ones. The "vulnerable persons" I am referring to here might either be younger patients who might have taken an overdose, or elderly patients who are extremely confused. People with learning difficulties are also fall into this category. This group I have drawn attention to is often well represented in our hospitals wards. The problems arise for many of these patients because when a confused patient is suffering from dementia, they will not understand why they are in hospital or indeed where they are at all. The hospital is not their home, or even their residential care home. Everything about it is different; the faces, the environment and the size. Basically it is an institution. It is no wonder they may exhibit confusing behavior when they might not know where they are or *why* they are there in the first place. When a person cannot easily remember even what happened a few hours ago, they might well get quite frightened when they find themselves in this alien environment. I have had many conversations with elderly patients who have gone from 'just' confusion into a more alarming paranoid state. Even the presence of the family is not always a comfort at this point.

Some vulnerable people will imagine all sorts of things. I have regularly been told by these people that their families have "put them there" or even that being in hospital is the result of a police conspiracy. In addition I have been informed in hushed tones by a number of these people that the family are after their money. It must be truly frightening not to have a firm grip on reality. It is not easy to listen to these fears and accusations (real or otherwise) in a helpful way. You do not want to collude with fantasy, nor do you want to disbelieve a real set of circumstances. I think I can safely say that this area presents a continuous learning curve for all of us in healthcare.

The point of mentioning this here is that this group of patients may be especially affected by issues of modesty, privacy and respect. It also brings up the subject of how we handle people when they are upset. They may be less aware in general of how they are looking to others, confused as they are. They may not notice when their bedclothes slide off the bed, or they may struggle with the practical and necessary encumbrance of oxygen masks, catheters and drips. It can be pitiful sometimes to see people whose dignity has been eroded in hospital. Stressed and understaffed wards are probably not the best environments for them, but the question is always, "where else?"

The confused state of mind of these particular patients affects others in the ward, too. Other patients suffer reactive distress at seeing the state of dress of vulnerable people. Furthermore, it is the more able minded who find it disturbing when a confused patient starts wandering. A number of patients will, during the course of their hospital stay, go "walkabout". It can look from their body language that they are 'on a mission'. These people have been known to try to get into bed with other patients, or go through their lockers or their handbags. Vulnerable patients make others vulnerable too. On many occasions I have found myself wheeling one of them round from leaving the perimeters of the ward back to their bedside. You can meet them from time to time in the corridors shuffling along with a fixed stare. Quite what they are searching for it is not clear, but I have a sense it may be for them, a "better place". The 'confused wanderer' does make life anxious for others however, both nursing staff and patient alike. Sometimes they can be more peripatetic at night than in the day. I am not sure that we have found the best way of handling this, though from time to time there have been instances of a 'tug of war' between the adjacent mental health facility and the acute hospital, each claiming that the other establishment is the right environment.

Patients will regularly explain to me how difficult this is to cope with. They can be both sorry for the other person and also a little fearful of what they might do next. Being targeted by another does little for a sense of safety whilst in hospital, and stress is inevitably caused by these experiences. Nursing staff continue to wrestle with the issue of vulnerable patients, knowing it would be better for all if there were other facilities for them. The same might be said for those who cry out all night, and sleep during the day. This is an invasion of privacy in another completely different way, but a reality on today's elderly and medical wards.

Not only the wanderlust patients but the noisy ones create distress for others. One long stay orthopaedic patient wrote to me recently of her experiences. "Unfortunately for me some of the things I have hardest to bear are being placed in a ward with 25 other patients. Many of those patients were suffering from dementia. For three weeks I was placed next to a woman who screamed at the top of her voice day and night without respite! I asked to be moved and was told that I had to be near a sink because of my infection. Finally after three weeks of lost sleep I felt some of my own resolve and determination weakening and I began to feel depressed."

PANIC STATIONS

It is not only the elderly who are vulnerable in this way. I was returning to the Chaplain's office one day when I came across a group of nurses attempting to restrain a clearly frightened and desperate patient. This person was perhaps in her forties, but she was getting very upset and the incident was spilling into the corridor where the general public was circulating. It did not look as if the presence of so many nurses was helping the situation. The woman was panicking. It was a bit like the heavy police presence at political rallies of different kinds that can spark off antisocial behaviour. What doesn't contain it might exacerbate the situation. Without thinking particularly I entered the fray as requested. I asked what the problem was, addressing the person at the centre of this melee as directly and calmly as possible. She told me that she did not want to go back to the ward. She thought that "they" were going to do something to her that she would not like. As the nurses were doing just that by restraining her with an over heavy presence it was creating more of a problem.

I asked the woman what she thought might help. She told me that she wanted her mother to come. That seemed very reasonable, particularly in the light of her panicky and anxious reaction to the restraint she was under. I then suggested that one of the nurses rang her mother so that she could be an advocate for her daughter and thus defuse a situation rapidly getting out of hand. When this was done and she was informed the woman then agreed to go back to the ward.

There might have been mental health issues present in that situation I don't know. However that is never an excuse for not asking a patient what might help them to be calm. It may be that some people have their panic buttons pressed by being in an institution in the first place, hospitals feeling like a foreign country to some. We cannot always know what peoples' backgrounds are, and those for instance who have had bad experiences in Local Authority Care homes may have justifiable overreactions to a heavy handed approach. It would remind them of some treatments from the past. Respect has to be given to all, irrespective of who we think they are or whether they are cooperating or not. In many cases a person familiar to the patient like a family member or a social worker may be all that is required to help a person feel more at ease in a hospital setting. Sometimes the presence of people in uniforms will prompt adverse reactions for various reasons, particularly among the vulnerable and fragile.

DIGNITY FOR ALL

Dignity may be described as a spiritual need too. To be given it is to be treated with respect and sensitivity and to be valued. It is a quality issue. Most patients are treated with dignity, and nine patients out of ten will tell you how the staff are wonderful. They will say things like "Nothing is too much trouble" and "They couldn't have treated me better". Praise indeed. Sometimes the media present a very different picture of hospital life. From my experience, the horror stories found from time to time in the media are very much in the minority.

Despite doing their very best for each patient in difficult circumstances, nursing staff may sometimes become over familiar with what they do, just as I might in my line of work. When they are confident in what they are doing because they have been practising it over time, it is easy for them to engage 'automatic pilot'. The danger of this is that it makes it easier to miss the symptoms of distress in patients. Physical distress will be addressed very quickly because often something practical can be done about it. It is less easy to cure emotional distress such as that presents when a patient is feeling threatened in a ward by the presence of unpredictable neighbours. In reality it cannot be sorted out satisfactorily. Life is not like that. It may take a long time to restore confidence to a distressed patient. It can however be understood by engaging them with understanding and empathy. Perhaps we best achieve this by putting ourselves in their shoes.

Having said that, we sometimes fail to recognise the vulnerability of nursing staff, who may be dealing with issues in their own lives that enter the ward experience, or they are simply overtired or overstretched. Doctors and nurses are people too, and from time to time they can experience their own traumas, burnout and ill health.

14

Spiritual care *is* quality care

When I speak of spiritual care and its relationship to quality care, it is not my intention either to suggest clinical or nursing staff are failing, nor for them to be loaded with yet more guilt, work and training. I believe though that we should expect some personal growth in the awareness of the many issues that relate to human need in a place of vulnerability. A hospital represents an environment where issues like respect, modesty and privacy do need to be protected. The giving of dignity and respect by others really do make people feel better about themselves. We always have to keep ourselves open to where these subtle pastoral insights are casualties to the more pressing practical tasks. It is not always a case of either performing one or the other. Exercising both good clinical and pastoral practice will surely help to bring a greater peace of mind to those for whom we care.

I was personally very grateful for the dignity and respect given me during a recent operation. When the time came for me to get on a trolley and be taken down to the pre-op room I was given a natty pair of special pants to wear. When my surgical gown flapped open, as they do, my modesty was happily preserved. When I had my first shower after my surgery, a nurse was present for my safety. It did not embarrass me particularly because she was not embarrassed. At times like this we have to be grateful for the professionalism of our hospital nursing staff, as it helps to get people back onto the road to recovery with the aid of respectful and gentle handling. That quality of care communicates that we are valued.

Principally, doctors have the upper hand psychologically, and their engagement with patients is very important. Other health care professionals, particularly the therapies are also in an excellent position to offer support to patients who are caused distress by lack of dignity or modesty and privacy issues. We can improve the attention we give to offer protection on the wards. Sometimes when nurses or physiotherapists listen carefully to people during the course of the other rehabilitation therapies they do, they may detect the wistful shadow passing over the person's face when speaking about the previous night or about other things going on for them on the ward. We can ask them to explain what they might have hinted at, and take them seriously. If anything can be done that would help it could be done. To listen is perhaps the best we can do. To understand this helps to give confidence and show that person that they are not alone. Any issues that need to be taken forward may be entered into the Kardex or patient notes. It is this total care that denotes quality in the engagement and foster restorative wellbeing to the patient.

It brings enormous encouragement simply to be heard. If that is the only thing we can do, I believe it is vital and it is supportive. As Sheila Cassidy writes; "Those who listen day after day in exposing themselves to another's pain are part of the healing process."(28) The worst place for anyone to be when things are happening to them which are beyond their control, is to be alone. To be listened to and understood, is not to be alone. How often we have been told, "Oh you *have* helped me," when all we have done is to be present and listen!

KEEPING A WATCHING EAR

When I had pneumonia and was rushed into St Bartholomew's Hospital in London thirty years ago with acute viral pneumonia, I was very ill. In the way people do, I really felt at one point I was going to die. My anxiety levels were very high at that time. In reality I was not going to die, but try to tell that to a person in a heightened state of anxiety and feeling less than rotten! One young nurse picked up the signals and made a point of seeing how I was before she went off duty. I cannot remember her name now or what she looked like, but she was like an angel to me at that point. How often do we hear this term 'angel' applied to nurses! You only need one person who takes an interest for the situation of 'bedside manna' to arise. Her care was a simple human connection in a frightening world of feeling awful, alien surroundings, regular injections and invasive doctor's rounds. As my condition was apparently "interesting" to the medical students according to the consultant, I was the ward guinea pig. It felt at the time a bit like Sir Lancelott Spratt from the Carry On series; but I wasn't laughing.

In my condition I could not fight them off, I was too fragile. That made me compliant. It was an overawing experience nonetheless. At least in all I was going through one member of staff recognised my humanity and responded appropriately to it. This was not rocket science to her but very effective spiritual care but flowed from who she was and I still remember it now. Someone reflecting on the level of compassion in healthcare, remarked that people did not usually remember what a person who had offered help and support actually said, what people remembered was that someone troubled to be there! Her interest represented quality to me. It addressed me as the person I was. It made a difference. As Ian McWhinney has commented, "In the end most people are healed by love". This observation is echoed by Sheila Cassidy who says, when talking of patients in a hospice, "If I were to sum up our pastoral care in the hospice, I would say we revealed to them that they are loveable." (29) Perhaps that is another name for spiritual care, a necessary quality in the ambient world of healthcare.

15

The trauma of spiritual pain and the "why" questions

Qaisra Khan who is spiritual and cultural care coordinator at Oxleas NHS Foundation Trust has observed: "People need to have their basic humanity acknowledged and respected. They also need in times of distress, to feel valued and to address the basic questions such as "why?"" (30) Finding meaning in our experience of ill health is a spiritual need.

People often ask "why" questions when bad things happen to them. What makes us feel fragile and bewildered is the illness that comes out of the blue, or the sudden accident or fall. Somehow people cannot reconcile these things with what they expected from life. It can easily bring them down and they may hit rock bottom and feel despairing. What I term spiritual pain or distress is often indicated by the "why" questions we ask, and occurs when our previous structure of life's meaning for us disintegrates as will often happen in illness. Spiritual pain is a component of any kind of pain, whether physical, mental or emotional and needs addressing as a potentially serious health issue. It is a focus of spiritual and holistic care. We have to learn to be aware of pain, emotional and spiritual and be sensitive to it. The opposite can also be true that if as an individual we have a grasp of the reasons why something is happening, we can be more resilient in the face of a crisis. As the psychoanalyst Carl Jung writes: "Suffering that is not understood is hard to bear, while on the other hand it is astounding to see how much a person can endure when he understands the why and the wherefore"(31)

So the experience is that people can stand suffering better if they can find a reason for it. Perhaps this is why you hear people say things like "Well, I am sure it is all for a purpose," or what is even more tragic, "God must mean me to learn something from this." These kinds of responses are often voiced I believe, largely because we do find it so difficult to accept the random way in which ill health can creep up on us. How many people have despairingly turned to me and asked, "Why has God done this to me; what have I done wrong?" Apart from a very bad press for God as vindictive, there are no ready answers to give. These comments represent a kind of defence mechanism though. Some truths are too hard to take all in one go; they need time. The doctor and priest, Gareth Tugwell and David Flagg ask the question "What does enable us to keep going against all the odds if there is not some sense of meaning or purpose?"(32)

In his book Theology and Joy, Jurgen Moltmann writes that "When a man sees the meaning of life only in being useful and used, he necessarily gets caught in a crisis of living, when illness and sorrow makes everything including himself seem useless."(33) It seems that apparently senseless suffering which persists but yields little discernible in the way of an end product somehow offends our sensibilities. It is as if "it just isn't cricket!" We just hate to be of no use. Illness creates this mirage. We believe it for a time and it incapacitates us. Our culture generally demands personal productivity and illness limits that. The feeling of uselessness that results also draws up spiritual pain. We may feel like a loser because we are not on top of things. "There must be some purpose for suffering" is a common feeling. When suffering catches us off guard there may be no time to prepare ourselves. We cannot gather ourselves for the impact to come. It just happens.

It is easier to bear something when we know what is to come. To be prepared is often very useful. For instance, when we hear a phlebotomist or nurse say "You'll feel a sharp prick" we can then prepare ourselves. We may also know that the short pain of an injection carries a meaningful outcome. There is a reason for the discomfort, and the blood results will assist the diagnosis or treatment. Some doctors will tell us that the treatment will hurt a bit, but it will not last long. I was told before an endoscopy, from a nurse who admitted me, "It's not very nice, though it only lasts a few minutes". I could then be ready for something uncomfortable but short lived. Though these preparatory statements will not make the physical pain any less, they may make the other experiences of pain manageable. We are prepared, so we need not be alarmed. The end product is probably worth the short

71

term discomfort. The warning of pain goes together with a desired outcome, for which it is worth enduring a little temporary pain.

WHY *NOT* ME?

The trouble is that in life 'bad things *do* happen to good people' - a phrase taken and amended slightly from a book about suffering. To take an extreme case, when a new born baby dies a short time after birth for no apparent reason, there is no way we can prepare for such a shocking and unexpected event. In the same way when a person has a fall at home despite being in sound health and mentally active, they are shaken up and dismayed. The consequence of the first example is emotional trauma, numbness and shock. In the second there is both a physical and emotional jarring to the whole system, a kind of total de-stabilisation. Both events however can be a kind of 'offence' to an imagined order of things that people have rightly or wrongly come to depend upon. Harry Williams says: " Even when the suffering is due to outward circumstance, like illness or catastrophe, it mauls as we have seen, the centre of our personal identity so that we suffer mentally and spiritually"(34) Hospitals are full of mauled people, not least those who may have to deal with long term incapacity including immobility, blindness and loss of speech.

For a young person, in some ways sudden ill health can be worse. When we are young we rarely contemplate mortality. The vibrancy of youth is a wonder to behold when the physical slowing of age and the sense of mortality gets to grips with you. One young person, Annabel Chown has described her experience of being diagnosed with cancer at the age of 31.

"I woke up in hospital on a beautiful May afternoon in 2002, aged 31 to be told that the seemingly benign cyst I'd just had removed from my left breast was actually cancer." She goes on in the article to describe the sudden change from summer into winter in her life. Shock and disbelief was gradually replaced by a kind of social isolation. It was as if she was plucked by an invisible hand out of a routine of life with certainties and independence, to a diminished and questioning person, existing in a kind of limbo.

She continued: "During my treatment and its aftermath, I completely lost my confidence as a woman although I was constantly complimented on my new "haircut" (a wig) and chemo-induced size-eight body. But I felt unattractive, invisible to men, and believed that most defining thing about me was my cancer. I felt it had taken over my life, cracked me open, ripped away the veneer by which I had previously defined myself – a successful career as an architect, long hair, a busy social life" (35)

For the bewildered young person or the more seasoned patient, spiritual pain is a reality, even if a person is unconscious of exactly what it entails for them consciously. All pain has a spiritual component whatever belief system a person possesses. The question of *why* is so often an accompaniment to these events and is itself an indicator of spiritual pain. "Why now?" people ask. Others will say "What have I done to deserve this?" or "Will I recover?" To these further questions others may arise like" What about my dog? " or "Where did it all go wrong?"

All questions like this need to be taken seriously, even when an answer isn't possible. Most of the time these questions, voiced or otherwise aren't always looking for answers, just a recognition of questions that have to be asked. These anxious queries have to be asked for the sake of our sanity. We have to somehow plot our journey through the experience. There are rarely any helpful answers. Spiritual care is more about taking those questions and the person who asks them *seriously*. We have to ask them. In the Bible, the Psalms which are part of wisdom literature are full of these 'why' questions. When others are around to share in the whys, the isolation of suffering may be alleviated.

SHOUTING AT DEAF SKIES

The diagnosis of life threatening disease has a profound effect on people who are ill and on their family and friends. Unsettling questions can often arise, such as "Why is this happening to *me?*" "What is the cause of this - is it my fault?", "How can I make sense of my condition?", and "How will I cope?". Many questions relate to identity and self-worth as patients seek to find an ultimate meaning in their lives."(38) These are all highlighted by the NICE Guidance on Cancer Services.

I hear these questions things regularly in hospital. While there are no simple answers to give people most of the time, it is often true that people are not looking for answers but validation of the questions asked and support in wrestling with them. These questions that indicate spiritual pain or distress commonly occur as a result of the damage caused to our particular pattern of beliefs or worldview. Most people want the world to be the shape they want it to be. We mostly try to control life. In today's world that is probably a luxury, as many millions are victims of the way the world is, whether in drought and war devastated countries, living under corrupt government or in the favelas of South America, shanty towns of South Africa as well as urban and rural areas of deprivation that exist in so many places.

We make up reasons as to why this unwelcome thing should happen or not and generally how we expect life to treat us. In this the world is probably filled up with optimists and pessimists, the 'empty glass and the glass half full' kinds of people. The 'whys' indicate that the person feels horribly let down by life. Feeling more like victims in the situation they feel kicked in the teeth by the unexpected. Behind the anguish and shock that accompanies sudden misfortune or the breakdown of health is a deep disappointment with the optimistic view of life that has kept us propped up in the past and has somehow inexplicably run out of gas. Where can we look for reassurance? It feels like no one is listening; the phone is off the hook. Ivan Mann has said that "when we are in affliction, our suffering is total. When life tears great gaps in our lives we should not try to fill them with words"(39) Holistic and spiritual care is about sharing the journey of pain more than about providing answers.

Spiritual pain or distress can take many forms. What each episode has in common is that it affects that sense of what it means for people to be human. It concerns people's deepest values and their meaning and purpose as persons in the world. Spiritual pain is known in experiences of disconnection, isolation, hopelessness, despair and guilt. These factors are experienced by people of faith and no faith. All value and meaning systems can collapse during ill-health, and this pain is deeply felt by all. In the Judeo-Christian tradition, the Psalms readily scream at God, life and circumstances.

This wisdom literature reflects the human condition and is undoubtedly borne out of very real everyday human situations when someone feels that God is far off. They are also echoes from a past age and culture for many of the "why" questions. The most quoted comes from Psalm 22; *"My God, my God, why have you forsaken me. Why are you so far from saving me, so far from the words of my groaning? O my God, I cry out by day, but you do not answer, by night and I am not silent."*(40) How many patients cry out; "Where are you in this Lord?" in the still watches of the night in hospital? The interesting thing is that even when people have little or no recognition of a higher power, the same kind of cry goes up.

THE GUILT OF ANGER

A case in point is the spiritual pain which affected Margaret, a woman in her late 60's. She had been suffering for some time with the deterioration of her lower leg after an operation. Whilst she was in hospital she had requested a visit from a chaplain. She was quite distressed, as her leg had become infected and the future looked bleak. She also had to cope with the physical pain of her arthritis. Everything that was happening to her created feelings of anger and bitterness in her and she was very confused. That is why she asked for a chaplain to visit.

When he arrived, he discovered that the issue of most concern to her was that she was very guilty about the anger she had towards God. Margaret was a woman whose faith meant a great deal to her. In her opinion God had let her down. The reason was that she felt that consenting to the operation, which she was fearful about in the first place, would help. But instead of getting better post-operationally she was getting worse and she was disappointed that God had not ensured success. Instead she felt cheated, let down and victimised by what was happening to her. Deep down she started to experience feelings of anger and resentment. As a result of having angry feelings Margaret then felt very guilty. She feared she might be losing her faith, which for her was the worst thing imaginable. It was then that she felt the need to talk to a chaplain. Bottling it up was only increasing her sense of isolation and fear.

When the chaplain arrived Margaret was clearly upset. As they had met before on the ward they were not strangers to each other. That helped them both to relax, and she came to the point immediately. Margaret shared her fear with him that she was losing her faith. When the chaplain asked her what made her feel that way, she unburdened herself about her anger towards God, who had 'let her down'.

Together they looked at her feelings. As they talked Margaret began to see that it might actually be very natural to feel that way in her circumstances, and that it was not *wrong*. He helped her see that no blame could possibly be attached to having feelings appropriate to what she was experiencing. Actually she only had to look at a few of the Psalms. Feelings only become wrong if we acted them out and deliberately caused pain or harm to other people. He explained to her that to feel anger was more a part of being fully alive than an indicator of a lack of faith. She asked for prayer, and felt a considerable amount of relief afterwards. It was like seeing things in a new way. The spiritual pain and distress somehow evaporated, and she no longer felt so isolated and despairing.

Shortly after that, Margaret had to undergo an amputation. Despite that she continued to feel a peace of mind that would have been unimaginable before. In subsequent visits she refers back to that conversation and the relief it seemed to bring. Again we go back to the difficulty of meaningless suffering. Her amputation was meant to enhance her life and not the opposite. The way in which she was helped to interpret her anger really seemed to affect her sense of wellbeing in a positive way. By being enabled to acknowledge and face up to her feelings for what they were, Margaret discovered a change in spiritual health and this appeared to affect her physically.

16

WE NEED OUR FEELINGS IN HOSPITAL

Spiritual care may be seen from Margaret's situation to be about the function of allowing people to have their very own natural and understandable feelings in a situation, and helping to contain them. It gives them back some autonomy in the situation. Margaret's was not an isolated incident. Experiences like this in hospital are happening all the time.

In the audit, or 'Minimum Data Set' that our chaplains fill in monthly to show our activity in hospital there is a recording item which is a specific indicator of spiritual pain. One of the entries is under 'Spiritual Healthcare Episodes'. On our weekly audit sheet, the definition of this 'Episode' is as follows: *A spiritual healthcare episode is an encounter where the person speaks of deeply personal or confidential matters, sheds tears, talks of death, God or asks for prayer or sacraments.*

In reality a large proportion of these encounters reported relate to spiritual pain resulting from the fact of illness, hospitalisation or a sudden and unexpected plunge into ill health. In terms of our mainstream ward visits, as opposed to the call-outs at night or via staff referrals during normal office hours, I believe the numbers of episodes are significant.

In 2006 with the paid chaplaincy staff we had 1079 spiritual healthcare episodes, and in the following six months, the paid staff encountered 969, and the chaplaincy volunteer visitors encountered another 330, making 1299 in all. This had risen to over 2500 in 2009. Considering that a patient was expressing here something very important to them, it was paramount that someone was there to take it seriously with open-ended time, allowing them to get it off their chest. In addition this kind of intervention that patients find so crucial is given recognition under the World Health Organisation's ICD coding for pastoral intervention (International Classification of Diseases):

"Pastoral Ministry (ICD code 96187-00) The provision of the primary ministry of presence and expression of the service, which may include:- establishing of relationship/engagement with another, hearing the story, and the enabling of pastoral conversation in which spiritual wellbeing and healing may be nurtured, and companioning/supporting persons confronted with profound human issues of death and dying, loss, meaning and aloneness." WHO 2002

As suggested at by the WHO definition, spiritual pain is also experienced as a kind of emptiness. For a believer in the Christian tradition this may be felt as God deserting them. It may be for others that life has let them down. The questions arise over what they can ever depend on again. Their previous comfort zones no longer provide peace of mind. This results in a kind of emotional vacuum or pathological Ground Zero experience. Some people, perhaps like Margaret will become very angry and look for someone or something to blame or hit out at. Others will take the anger upon themselves and become isolated within themselves. This makes them very hard to reach. In the health service we have to take this issue of spiritual pain very seriously because it is all around us. It is a profoundly difficult thing to face losing one's health, or suffer an accident. Very little may stay the same when our life has been interrupted but such a cruel and uninvited visitor.

Our hospital staff regularly experiences the presence of spiritual pain. They may not be aware of exactly what they are encountering or attach this description to it. However, when our staff members have been called into intensive care wards or the maternity ward to be with staff, this is often what is happening. When a number of baby deaths occur, especially stillbirths, the staff who are on the particular shift in which this unusual series of events occur can find themselves hitting a caring 'wall' like the marathon runner. In the intensive wards this may happen also when a patient who has been there for a long time, picks up and seems to be making a good recovery when he suddenly dies. It affects the staff. There are emotional attachments. There is a sense of failure. The 'why' questions will arise in this context too, along with the feeling "This shouldn't happen, should it?" These thoughts may be accompanied by the unconscious question "Where have we failed?" In these situations is as if both the personal and the professional aspects of staff members become deeply challenged by events. A feeling of despair can readily set in with resulting inertia. It then becomes hard to get on with the job as if nothing has happened. The same questions arise when a member of staff dies suddenly. "This is wrong" is the unconscious feeling among colleagues.

WHAT DOESN'T SEEM *RIGHT*

From time to time nursing or medical staff do die. Being on the 'right' side of the sheets, as the term goes, we do not expect it. Again, a corporate atmosphere kind of spiritual pain arises, because hospital staff will often feel unconsciously that they are the carers and the ones they look after are the sick ones. They are there to work to make the patients better, how can staff then die? It is an illogical position to take, but it is there. When a medical team member dies, it is more likely that they will be remembered for a long time afterwards, for along with the usual feelings of grief and loss, there is also the sadness and anger which is generated by the gap left. The impossible has happened and suddenly the world has lost its old familiar meaning and shape. Even the deceased member can become targeted as letting their colleagues down. "Why didn't they say they were not feeling well?" "We were just beginning to gel as a team, and now it's all gone to waste." Sometime staff can turn this grief in on themselves and blame themselves for what has happened. They may desperately try to look for adverse health indicators in that person that they may have missed before they died.

A recent item of news that has hit the headlines a few years ago which exemplifies the shock and disbelief that often lies behind the feeling of spiritual pain that people feel. A three year old girl called Madeleine McCann was abducted from her bedroom in an otherwise safe holiday environment in the Algarve, while her parents had a meal a short distance away. They took it in turns to check on her and her younger siblings every few minutes. She was fair haired, pretty and full of life. Despite intensive publicity and international police activity she has not been found, and no one implicated in her abduction. To add salt to her parents' wounds, they themselves found that the finger of suspicion was pointed at them by the local police based on evidence that seemed very flimsy It was so slender that it could be construed quite differently both by prosecution and defence lawyers. They then became formal suspects. Thankfully the suspicions were dropped but their daughter has never been found. I cannot begin to imagine what spiritual pain factor remains central in their lives even years later.

The Daily Telegraph ran an article one week after her disappearance that echoed what we have often repeated in our Staff Induction training on Cultural and Spiritual Awareness. The article was entitled "Misplaced trust that led to Madeleine's betrayal." The article makes a case for the risk element to be factored into all that we do these days. "Terrible things happen, but we trust that they are not going to happen to us." (39) We trust that the world is a relatively safe place. Madeleine's parents trusted that the resort facilities were perfectly safe, and Madeleine as a small child would have had implicit trust in her parents to keep her safe. Tragically none of this happened. Madeleine's parents now have to trust the police and the vigilance and good will of the public, but today the trail has gone much colder. Whatever happens, a long dark cloud had been cast over that summer for many people, the "why" questions will go on being asked; the different circumstances in which spiritual pain arises will persist. I am sure that for the McCanns the feeling of outrage will be there among the rest.

The newspaper article does not apportion blame. It simply highlights the fact that the unbelievable *does* happen. Moreover it can happen to you or me. So shocking is this fact that, if we are honest, none of us is prepared for it, and that we have to find coping mechanisms to deal with it. The reality is this is that is the kind of world we live in and not any other more sanitised version. Children get abducted, adults and babies even hospital staff die unexpectedly, and we become ill and have accidents. We probably cannot change this, but we can learn to share the darkness with each other, even if we are unable to "make it better." For medical staff whose lives are dedicated to making things better this is particularly hard to bear. This sharing of the spiritual pain does not come easily; it is a feeling to be learned. It is an art more than a science. Often it is those people who appear to have been dealt a poor hand of cards in life who seem to be better able to respond in these situations. As the humorous quote on our chaplaincy notice board once read; "Blessed are the cracked, for they are the ones who let in the light." We know we cannot heal the wounds associated with traumatic and sudden happenings or prolonged ill health with words, but we can learn. These people often do find the way to do it with an understanding and compassion born of their own wounds.

Among the many caring and empathetic people working in our health service will be those who recognise that the patient's presenting symptoms do not tell it all. They have come to understand that beneath exteriors which may range from stoic and defiant to broken and depressed, are important feelings that need to be both expressed and heard. I would hope that chaplains are very experienced in this kind of spiritual care which supports people in these moments. In addition the porter, the domestic assistant as well as the nurse and clinician who may know spiritual pain first hand, also have a considerable part to play.

17

THE CRY OF THE TRAUMATISED HUMAN HEART

Many situations in healthcare develop to reach a stage no one wants. But do we always discern the hidden depths of the sufferer when the unwished for happens? Does our healthcare service normally extend to those depths? The deterioration that many experience when ill may actually be exacerbated by hospital surroundings that seem strange, and also the manner in which attention is given to them. A case in point happened when the author Cristina Odone's father hit rock bottom during a recent illness, and like others I have frequently met just did not want to go on, if going on meant 'more of this'. She describes the situation when pressure was put on her to cooperate with him in accelerating his decline. "Yet now he wanted out. I could see that what would kill him faster than any disease was the realisation that he was dependent on unsympathetic strangers, and stuck in a disorientating and unfamiliar place: he felt humiliated, vulnerable and out of control. But I didn't want to kill him. I wanted to kill the men and women around him who were failing so manifestly in caring for him. If they had been doing their job properly, they could have controlled his pain, treated him with respect, even maybe engaged with him to raise his spirits. My father didn't need assisted suicide, he needed assistance." (40)

People who become ill or are involved in life changing situations, such as having a stroke or a head or spinal injury, are still people who have feelings. They have not chosen this turn of events in their lives. All kinds of conflicting feelings will arise to compromise their adjustment to and acceptance of their situation as well as their rehabilitation. Alongside all the excellent research, technology and supportive medical interventions that the medical profession can provide there remains a need also for real understanding and support of the wounded self at the heart of these people.

WHEN THE GOING GETS TOUGH...

You cannot but admire the resilient human spirit. Over the past decade I have been privileged to see many people who have undergone life changing experiences that have come upon them unbidden and left them a vestige of their former selves. Despite this they have fought back and carved out a new life for themselves. Among these people have been the spinally injured. This kind of injury may have happened to them in an accident, a microsecond of inattention, or as a result of an illness that has affected the spinal cord. Sometimes unfortunately, it has been as a result of an operation which has left them in that way.

Other people who seem to have risen above their situations of difficulty are those who have been badly burned. Some have been burned because of a domestic argument that went very sour, while others have been burned as a result of an industrial accident. Quite a number who end up in Burns Units are those with learning difficulties. Some of them have not always been able to handle the finer points of cooking incorporating risks that boiling liquids, or the management of gas hobs present. However many victims of burns have survived these traumas and proceeded to master the specific disabilities that this kind of accident can bring about. The first burns patient I ever met was suffering as the result of a domestic dispute that got out of hand. I wonder how many different layers of healing were required in that instance?

There are less sensational reasons for life changes that will come into effect through illness and trauma to the brain, but which nevertheless require radical new departures in life. Strokes and illnesses like Guillain-Barre Syndrome (a disorder affecting the peripheral nervous system, often resulting in temporary paralysis) and head injuries sustained in countless ways take people back to new beginnings. These are totally unexpected and unasked for but which require great courage and the support of others to face. The desire of people to work through the shock and depression that follows such events can only draw admiration from us. They seem to know for the most part that they have to come to terms with the questions "what if" and "if only", and set their face to move on and recover skills that have been wiped out very suddenly. None of this is easy. There are many tears and dark periods on the way.

THE HEALING OF TIME

The temptation of health care to become a kind of biological garage and thus to adopt a task- centred 'fix-it' culture is, in the light of financial stringency and the pressure of number, overwhelming. It is also understandable. However it needs to be pointed out that healing takes time, whether for the body or the mind. There is too much of the 'instant' in our 21st Century culture anyway. It is seductive, and we should know when to resist it and be counter culture.

Over the years I have found myself saying to stroke patients who have lost the capacity to speak, that they may feel in a strange country at present. I may go on to say that with time and patience they will be surprised what improvements they may be able to make. With a massive stroke usually communication is almost impossible, and recovery a lot less likely. This may be small consolation to people, and I could be criticised for giving untutored hope. My experience is that many stroke patients rarely stay in the same place physically as they are immediately after a stroke but move on with improvement in communication and motor skills. I think many are relieved that someone other than nursing staff bothers to address them in this in-between state.

Physiotherapists and Occupational therapists, along with nursing staff are familiar with the support these people need, and make sure they aid any improvements are possible. Families who attend less frequently than staff can also communicate to them as they can 'read' them better than people who do not know them so well. Stroke patients are grateful if you treat as the *person* they are. This is one of the kindest supports we can give. It is spiritual care of the highest order when we give back dignity to the person who has seemingly lost everything through a stroke.

I regularly witness immense courage in people like this. Almost without being prompted people will look forward and not back under these circumstances. With all the conditions listed above, looking over the shoulder at the past is like staring into a cul-de-sac. There is nowhere to go. Many people from the spinally injured to the brain injured will tell you "You just have to get on with things". It is heartening to see people in their later years doing their exercises to build strength and struggle with words to communicate as if life depended on it, which of course for them it does. But it takes time.

In one way our lives do depend on addressing the challenges before us. It is so easy to go under when we concentrate on lamenting what has happened to us. The experience of grief is natural at the loss of faculties, and indeed, the loss of an earlier 'life'. To look forward and focus on recovery is the way ahead and that is precisely why so many people living with a changed life do it. The degree to which people re-invent themselves is astonishing. The Spinal Injuries Gym enables people to gain sporting skills and muscle tone sometimes in a way that they did not before they were affected by an injury. If we look at this cynically we might call it compensation, but in another way it is a commendable recycling of energy and focus to become something other than simply a *disabled person*. Perhaps the insights developed by people who may only have months to live apply equally to those having to face change in this way. "People deal with such news differently, some never come to terms with it. But most go through an acceptance process that includes anger and disbelief, but ultimately leads them to re-evaluate life." (41)

THE HEALING OF 'NORMALISATION'

Strange happening can bring people into hospital just as much as a slow deterioration or a viral infection or more predictably an elective surgical operation. I heard from one person that the reason they broke their spine was they stepped backwards to admire some handiwork and tripped over a low wall. It was as easy as that. The resultant spinal injury was to change that person's life totally. Others had a viral infection that resulted in a condition, such as Guillain-Barre syndrome that rendered them totally paralysed. One person told me that in ICU they heard people talking about them, but they could only see them but not talk or gesticulate back. What a truly frightening experience this was. That person made a full recovery. One young girl told me how she had no feeling at all in her legs and she was horrified to find that she could not stand, but when I came across her it was slowly returning. Others with the same illness were not so fortunate and were quite disabled by it. Whatever the outcome, the whole experience was profoundly scary. Some of the support groups and charities involved were really targeted on effective support by having past sufferers in their team. These people could understand the 'territory' that the present sufferers were lost in, and this helped the normalising of people in what had begun as highly abnormal. You could describe these support groups as 'fellow travellers'.

Many people were admitted over the years in our orthopaedic wards as a result of Road Traffic Accidents. One particular surgeon in one of our Trust's hospitals would sometimes give me a ring when I was a chaplain there to ask me visit people who were suffering flashbacks after RTA's. I would begin by going into these encounters a bit blind, but over time I was drawn into acquiring some training in trauma counselling. In the event would always let the patient describe to me what their experience was. They would often be very scared and felt that they might be a bit odd as the event repeated itself regularly for days or weeks after the accident.

I was able to tell them that it was very normal to experience flashbacks. This is when the incident or aspects of it replayed itself like a film in a person's consciousness (or even when asleep). Sometimes though it felt like a real physical experience; something shocking. It was understandably scary to people when this happened. Usually is a phenomenon that decreases with time. For those with Post Traumatic Stress Disorder, where the experience undergone was sudden, traumatic, unexpected and involved personal responsibility or loss of life, the experience can create problems over many years. The World War I notion of 'shell shock' is about this very thing.

It was good in my situation to inform people of that waning effect, and that yielding to the flashbacks was better than trying to 'fight them', if indeed you could. I suppose the experience is similar to a particular vivid dream that repeats, but with added feelings of panic. But it is still very real and frightening.

There is something about the speed at which these accidents occur, that imprints moving image on the 'CCTV' of one's mind. Others on the other hand could not remember anything just before the impact. Again there was nothing strange about this; it happens. The accident victim's experience is just another way in which traumatic events are processed. This could be made to feel more normal when people are told that it is an experience shared by many. To go through these things on your own is bad enough, but to think that you are abnormal because of the repercussion or indeed the absence of recall adds another dimension of worry. To try to explain that these are abnormal experiences happening to normal people can help the unease to lessen. Families can be understandably anxious themselves and they can contribute a bit of shock and anxiety to these circumstances. The attempt to 'normalise' people is about the principle of containing. Containment helps a person to come to terms with things, and know that they are not strange but par for the course.

Even the event that on outward inspection seems tragic, can in some circumstance bring a kind of healing through the process of getting back to normal. One of the most curious examples of this kind of experience came in the lives of two people who suffered from a genetic disorder. As a couple they naturally yearned for a family. Their family tried to put them off, as indeed did the clinicians, knowing as they did about the genetic probabilities of abnormalities. Nature had its way however and they did have a child, who was eventually born dead. The physical abnormalities differences were evident. I was called in at night to the Maternity ward say a blessing for the baby as the couples had requested, and met up for the second time with them. The first meeting was not an easy one for they were understandably very angry with God for their condition and the further deprivation of not being able to have children themselves.

When I entered their room I dreaded what I might meet but I found them were smiling and relaxed. The baby was in a small Moses basket, quite pitiful to see. We chatted on about the fact of who the baby most looked like and about other baby related matters. The reason for their incongruous pleasure at the time then became clear to me because now they felt they were 'normal'. They had a *baby*, albeit one that had not survived - just like anyone else. They could talk about the baby and experience a very natural occurrence. For this couple even the grief was something that linked them to other people they knew. They did not feel like outsiders to ordinary life. Despite the sadness there was a measure of *normalisation* here that made them feel very human.

Humour; the Oil in the Machine

The place of appropriate humour in the whole business of recovery and rehabilitation cannot be underestimated. It is for some people the way to come to terms with bad things that happen. Certainly among the elderly who have been through the privations of war you seem to find a "Dunkirk Spirit" and ability to laugh at themselves. A person who recently experienced a blue light trip to hospital highlighted the necessity for seeing the lighter side in a letter he wrote shortly after he was discharged. He said "This of necessity played an important part. With patients, who by virtue of their accidents suffer huge trauma, humour is an essential element within the given care; between staff, staff with patients and between patients".

In the Hospital grounds we have had a prefabricated building not unlike a temporary classroom that you see in many school playgrounds. In this the Head Injuries Support Group, known as Second Chance was housed. It has since moved to the heart of Wakefield. It acts as a Day Centre and a support group to many in the area. Here a group of people who had had different kinds of head injuries come on different days to do activities, meet socially and be part of an extended family. It is managed by staff who have had to learn over time how to relate to and care for people with brain injuries. Here there is an atmosphere of busyness and endeavor as well as laughter and the inevitable jokes at each other's expense. For them this seems to oil the wheels of managing the life changes and the mixed nature of getting on with things. People at Second Chance have all arrived via several routes, car accidents, brain tumors and cerebral haemorrhages to name a few. The atmosphere is very harmonious for the most part, as the people are able to settle down confident that they are among the like-minded, fellow travellers who have each experienced a head injury that has changed them.

Despite the accumulated bad luck stories that constitute the histories of its clients, Second Chance has been one of the most positive places to be in the hospital. This is surprising because many of the users have trouble communicating verbally, some are physically disabled and others suffer memory loss. Everyone seems to be accepted for the personalities that they are. Rather than lamenting their situation in life they attempt to grow into the "new" them. They also represent differing age groups, social backgrounds and academic abilities. They are a family. Some have published books about how their life has changed, others will tackle woodwork or make Christmas Cards, while others will play snooker or dominoes. There is a "school" timetable in the week and on one morning there will be a mathematics emphasis and on another that of English grammar or comprehension. It works.

Whilst no one would wish ill health or accident upon anyone else, there is often a defining moment in recovery. I shall mention the watershed experiences people have in other parts of this book, but I cannot help but being reminded of Ralph Waldo Emerson's words: "We forget ourselves and our destinies in health, and the chief use of temporary sickness is to remind us of these concerns." (42)

People are dynamic entities not static. We are born, grow and develop through our life learning, experiences and battles and hopefully through them learn how to become. As the saying goes, "What doesn't kill you makes you stronger." Illness viewed in this way can be a part of our education, because it reminds us of our mortality on the one hand, and the preciousness of each moment of life on the other. It reminds us that we need each other, our stories, our interdependence and our humour, provided it is not in bad taste or mere facetiousness.

18

THE TRAUMA OF COLLATERAL DAMAGE

To use a well worked phrase, when one suffers all suffer. What happens to us affects those around us in many different ways. From emotional "fall-out" to the extra practical work that may be involved when a friend or relative is sick, others around feel the effects.

"Pebbles in the pool" is the catch phrase introducing a section of a new DVD presentation made on by the hospital based Brain Injuries support unit Second Chance, described in the last chapter. They know the ripple effect of trauma because those around the affected person feel the impact of their condition. When trauma occurs there will be those ripples that eventually reach the furthest point from the pebble's initial splash. In a similar way sickness affects the whole circle of life. Relationships, employment, leisure pursuits and how and where we live can all fall victim to illness. It probably most affects the people closest to us. This ripple effect determines the way that people see and experience themselves, their loved ones, and their ambitions hopes and fears in life. Patterns of living can be halted or disrupted by illness or changed forever. Peoples' view of life, and meaning, even the concept of a higher power gets caught up in the experience that bad health brings upon them. This is all part of the package present in the patient that carers, professional and otherwise, may encounter when providing support.

Some time ago I was phoned at work by a woman with whom I had been professionally involved for some years. My association with her family covered care in the hospital for her husband, a funeral, a memorial service, a 'one year on' remembrance and eventually a new marriage. She and her family, particularly her mother, Betty would come along to chapel on Sundays on a regular basis until they moved slightly further away to their roots so that the whole family would once more be together. A second phone call followed only a few weeks later in which this woman informed me that her mother had contracted a serious and aggressive neuro-physiological disorder. On this particular day the message was that Betty had gone downhill very quickly, and could I come. All plans had changed, and from nursing her at home, the family was told by Betty that she wanted to go to a hospice where everything would be purpose adapted, and her own family would not have to suffer the inconvenience of 24 hour care.

The ripples in this pool were very much in evidence when I arrived at the house. There were tears, numerous cups of coffee, constant phone calls and the door bell ringing as Macmillan nurses, district nurses and others finished their tasks or dropped by to make assessments for the next stage of disability. It was all about shock and sudden change. Everyone was busy caring and thinking of Betty, but the emotional undertow was also present in the room. The speed of the onset of illness appeared to be just too much for everyone, and they hardly had time to deal with their strong feelings. From the dream of moving to their new location to enjoy their declining years this elderly couple had to face huge loss along with all their family.

When I arrived, Betty, having been helped to bathe and make herself presentable to me 'her surprise guest', was wheeled into the room and carefully placed in her chair. She glowed with a peace and radiance she had no right to in the circumstances, but then she was always that sort of person. In her working life, Betty had been involved in social work, so she was aware of how nurses tied in with carers and the doctor, and she was allowing it to all happen round her. After nearly an hour with the whole family the two of us had a treasured moment alone. It was a little chat and a prayer as I held her hand. There was a bond of knowing that happens sometimes, when the truth is never spoken but somehow *known*. Both before and after that moment the rest of the family were both rallying round her, preparing for the move to a hospice and carrying inside themselves the possibility of their lives changing. Her sudden condition had affected everybody. Their hopes for the future had to be revisited. Questions of fairness were being asked. Few answers were forthcoming. Betty died soon after. That was another ripple for the family to live with.

DREAMS FADE

We all have dreams. We hope that life will pan out for us in a certain way. Some dreams are a bit hopeful, even a bit fantastic. Other hopes or dreams are very possible to achieve and with some hard work and good fortune they may well materialise. The person for instance who wants to be a nurse and shows gifts of caring, efficiency and concern for the welfare of others is likely to achieve their goal, provided they satisfy the various panels and university departments. All along they will encounter professionals who will assess their suitability and whether they satisfy the academic standards required.

When a person becomes ill, it is very hard for them to maintain such dreams or plans for the future. Somehow their hopes become thwarted by illness, and the present experience seems to have a limiting effect upon thoughts of a present let alone a future. As with the terminally ill this can change a person's whole view of life. People deal with it differently. When people come into hospital it is so important to hear their story, should they want to tell it.

In a BBC News article recently a patient described the effect of knowing that each day is precious and it can alter one's value system. A man who was diagnosed with Hodgkins Lymphoma, a cancer that affects the whole lymphatic system spoke as he reflected on the materialism of his life when healthy: He said that "None of these material things really matter, illness demolishes them all." Seeing that illness changes our perspective, this same man discovered new sense of focus, commenting further; "However awful, tedious and catastrophic being terminally ill may be." The dulling effect of ill health can be described for some people as an experience that turns one's personal world from technicolour to monochrome.

This diminishing of personal aspiration will depend of course upon the severity of their condition, and the mindset of the individual. A person coming into hospital for routine surgery will usually have no such worry. Their dreams and plans might embrace hopes of much better times ahead. A fit and well person is unlikely to entertain any thought of limitations upon their lives. The world, as it is said is their oyster. For these people everything seems possible and the sky is the limit for the future. For the fit or recently recovered, holidays may be planned, projects undertaken and even challenging mental and physical targets like a higher degree or the London Marathon may be anticipated. After routine surgery children and young people, providing they are reasonably healthy anyway, will put their health experience aside and think all things are possible. The skies are always seeming blue for these people and in their general mindset of energetic optimism bad weather rarely threatens!

STORM CLOUDS

One of the problems with physical illnesses or major operations is that they cast a shadow over almost every aspect of life. The person undergoing a hip or knee replacement is going to view their next holiday differently from before. The issues of mobility and the suitability of the destination for someone not quite as sprightly as before will have to come into the picture. This is actually very prudent. It would be unsuitable or even dangerous to tackle Lake District fells when operating at a lesser capacity than before. Life will have to change. Certain losses may have to be faced for the first time like dropping a physical activity or hobby because of the decrease in physical aptitude.

It is not all bad news. I was very surprised when looking at a manufacturer's website extolling the virtues of metal to metal hip replacements with a video featuring one successful post- operative patient fell running and another doing aerobics classes as if life after the operation was better than before! I felt that this scenario might only apply to a small minority and may have been misleading for the majority of people. However in defence of these particular claims (made by the manufacturer of prosthetics) some patients *will* actually rejoice in new found mobility and freedoms to exercise that they have not experienced for years. Certainly many people will testify to the wonderful new lease of life that they experience when they have a joint replacement that eliminates pain altogether.

These orthopaedic procedures are actually at the more positive end operational interventions. There are other operations and other conditions that clip our wings very much more dramatically. The

94

effect of post illness or operational change on people come can herald the appearance of dark clouds on the horizon. The recognition of our health limits alters the way in which we reflect on our lives. I have regularly heard quite elderly people say with pride that they have been able to visit their children in Canada or Australia in the past, and wistfully comment that they do not think that they will be doing that again. This represents quite a savage loss, and we wonder quite how those people will manage that loss. Is this recognition of their mortality and the winding down of activity that once they undertook without a second thought? If so is the addressing of this loss a health care issue. Surely these holistic considerations form part of that patient's psychological, emotional and spiritual need. We who work within the spiritual and pastoral care department would say a resounding "Yes." It may even be that the shared and supported understanding of their difficulty of facing deprivations, may lead to a greater degree of vitality to invest in their remaining years.

ONE SIZE FITS ALL?

One aspect about people that is inescapable in health care is the variation of individual temperaments and general spirit. Some elderly people will display an indomitable defiance in the face of adversity, and treat their physical decline with humour and resolution. One woman I knew was courageously facing complex respiratory difficulties, and had test after test with no clear result. When in fact she did have some news it was not at all good, and she was told she had cancer. Almost immediately she declared that she wanted to go to a particular hospice some miles from her home, and once there died before I could get to visit her. Other people seem to see hospitalisation and illness as a temporary irritation or annoying disruption to the process of living.

One elderly stroke patient I saw had been readmitted for the third time in the past year, each time representing a further deterioration in her physical state. When I saw her recently she was describing the tingling in her legs that she put down to the vigorous physiotherapy session she had that morning. She proudly announced that one of the physiotherapists had said to her "Oh you are a real star; a real go-er;

I wish there were others like you." You could see what pleasure she was getting from these appreciative remarks about her willingness to give her all in order to get out of hospital and proceed with her life. Other patients are only too keen to continue leisure pursuits such as ballroom dancing, which seems to be an interest that is followed with vigour by extremely elderly people. You have to admire the differences in people, particularly in those who will not be halted by a temporary bout of ill health!

19

THE TRAUMA OF FALLING; THE LAST STRAW?

Orthopaedic wards in hospitals are often termed 'Orthopaedic Trauma' for obvious reasons. One moment you are putting up the washing and the next you are on the ground with a broken hip. You go out for the newspaper or the milk, and you do not see the black ice and . . . whoops, before you know it you have broken wrist. Then you are on your way to A&E before you can mentally process the experience.

One of the frequent situations I come across is that of the elderly who have a fall. These people may be victims of accidents in their home or garden or down at the Shopping Centre. Others fall when on holiday abroad and are flown home for treatment. It is usually quite a shock, particularly if it has never happened before. I often hear the comment, "It's just not like me," or "I really don't know what happened." Many people will say that they felt so foolish to have a fall, as if the fact of it automatically placed them in a category of 'fallers'. Most people will be mildly traumatised, and spend some days thinking back on the moment and trying to work it out. Apart from the treatment of the inevitable fractures, once in hospital further tests will be carried out looking at indicators such as blood pressure, neurological problems, anaemia and brain conditions. In my opinion, patients need an equal amount of support for what I term *destabilisation*. When a person has a fall out of the blue, they can often become physically and emotionally shaken up, irrespective of the reason for the fall. This sudden turn of events can make life go topsy- turvy for a few days. Often this followed by a loss of confidence. A fear invariably enters that person's head that it will happen again once they are fit to walk again. Even getting mobile can take longer because of lowered muscle tone and a loss of confidence. This is very common, and as listeners we need to understand that it is a scary time and our consistent support needs to be given also to the non-physical aspects of the consequences of having a fall.

Once a victim of a fall has been assessed there will be a recovery time in hospital. This does not often take long; but it depends. We have to remember that if a person breaks a hip, it would take six to eight weeks to heal by natural means. Unless this is a hairline fracture which will heal under bed rest and gentle movement, this is not the usual way. A break at the femoral head, a common fall fracture, needs an effective, long term solution. Instead a hip replacement is carried out which can mean that the recovery time is more like two weeks at the most. During this time is spent healing and trying to gain some mobility. Patients will not always understand the reasons for the delay in returning home, and anxiety may set in. The keen interest of occupational therapists surrounding the suitability of your home is difficult to understand when you have lived there for twenty or thirty years with no problem. The realisation may then dawn that life will change and that all these arrangement are trying to help the person to avoid another fall. This is another example of the ripples in the pool; that a fall may herald the fact that life will never be the same again.

EMOTIONAL TRANSITIONS OF RECOVERY

From a medical and therapeutic point of view all these provisions for future safety are important. Emotionally though, it is a lot for an elderly person to take in. The health professionals involved with that person intend to work with them to enable them to eventually gain independence. The feeling a patient is left with however may one of being unnecessarily 'nannied' when they don't want it. At this point in the rehabilitation there may be tensions between the patient and the health service. As well as necessary new arrangements in the home, it may also be that a Care Package needs to be put in place. This is most likely when a person lives alone, or has little family support. This means that Care Assistants may come in to help the person out of bed and bathing in the morning, check on lunch provision at midday and be here for evening meal or getting them to bed. It does make some independently minded people feel as if they are being treated as children, and it is not difficult to see how they may resent it. However, it only happens after clear assessment, and it is for the person's good.

It may feel like the beginning of the end. It is certainly experience as a loss of independence, and we need to recognise the debilitating effect of this upon a person's spirits. Every 'loss' needs to be recognised and taken seriously, even if there is nothing that can be done to avoid it. It takes us back to the erosion of power, and really that some emotional support needs be be provided there to enable independently minded people come to terms with the changes.

The final blow to independence after a fall might be that the assessment might prompt the person's family to start on the process of suggesting some kind of residential care for their relative. This stage of the process graphically illustrates the way things change after an unplanned hospital stay later on in life. It also shows how a time in hospital may serve as a watershed experience for the elderly as well the young. The younger person may recover only to try to amend their lifestyle, or gain a better insight into what is important in life. On the other hand the elderly person be experiencing what seem like a cruel change in circumstances that was not anticipated even a few months before. It may seem like the downward path. It certainly requires a pause for reflection and the contemplation of possible future plans and choices, particularly if their mobility is compromised or independence threatened. The gentle trauma and distress in this whole scenario is because a person's meaning, identity and purpose in life are questioned by these changes. Because of that the issues around these changes are as emotional and spiritual as they are practical.

ALTERING *MY* HOME

A more radical development in the scenario of repeated falls may finally indicate that things will have to change in the home to keep that person safe. We have already touched on the need for adaptations, so the person can get around more easily, especially if a wheelchair is needed. Not only does a fall affect joints and bones, it can destabilise a person's general health. Patients often say how much they feel shaken up by a fall, and that their confidence to walk again has diminished. When you link this experience up with the resultant loss of muscle tone that affects all elderly people who have been bed bound for a week or two, you have a recipe for very slow recovery. Some people never make the journey back to full mobility. Much of the work of physiotherapists in the acute setting is around the task of getting elderly people to walk again. At the same time the person's home is assessed for suitability. As mentioned before the occupational therapist's task is to make that assessment. If they live on their own it may be that certain aids and alterations like handrails and bathroom adaptations are required to help that person get about more easily. All this takes time and can cause the length of hospital stay to increase. As a result of all these things the time may come for independent living to be abandoned for the safer environment of residential care. That sudden loss of independence is a bitter pill to people swallow. It may signal for them an 'end of life' path. It will most certainly draw up feelings of great loss. Much of our support for patients is in the area of this particular life change. It is heartrending to see the dawning realisation in some people that they will never be back in their own homes. The future to them seems fraught with uncertainty and tinged with loss. As we know it isn't the end; it can be just the beginning of a new stage of life.

WEIGHING RISKS

The risk factor is taken very seriously by those involved in the discharge of patients. There are certain tests against which the suitability for independent living is assessed. Sometimes people are simply too weak to go back to the home that they have left without the risk of another fall, domestic accident or self- neglect through functional disability. Some people are ready to see this and reluctantly accept the consequences, while others just cannot accept it and fight all the way to the Residential Home. To accept the need to go into residential care can be the point of recognition that your life may be on the wane from what it had been. Even if things turn out differently, it can really hurt.

Where there are others around who are able to support, there is a measure of safety and security. Where there are not there is a serious risk factor in emotional destabilisation. Families can play a very important part here in the gentle persuasion that is sometimes required. Where it is not handled sensitively, it can bruise relationships. It certainly cannot be rushed. The members of the hospital staff are often aware of these dynamics, but may not have the time to stay with the slow and painful process of adaptation. Those with more open ended time may well find they have a valuable opportunity to allow people to come round in their own time.

I met a woman in a rehabilitation ward some years ago, who after the first few minutes of conversation invariably brought the conversation round to a certain topic. She would express genuine surprise and upset that her son had put her house on the market, and the family had got together to 'put her in a home.' As a regular ward visitor, seeing maybe hundreds of patients between repeat visits, it was hard to keep track of the sequence of events that she was describing. Her deep concern about what was going on was not in doubt. In these days when the needs of the vulnerable adult have come to the fore, it is relatively simple to raise concerns with the ward staff. They may then check it out and refer on the Social Worker if necessary. The questions I was asking myself were whether this person had misunderstood her family's real intentions, and whether they have they really communicated together over this significant decision? Personally, I could not make up my mind about the matter, and just listened to her worries. I think perhaps in the circumstances I might have more proactive and referred on the matter to others. There is always a danger of sticking your nose in or even colluding with someone who has completely misunderstood a situation. Maybe they have become slightly paranoid about things. Reflecting positively on this situation however, sometimes the children just want their elderly parent to be safe. They may feel them to be too vulnerable or unsafe at home. Sometimes they live too far away or busy to keep an eye on their welfare or act as front line carers. It is not always sinister, and often done "for the best." The stress caused was also significant; a matter that required recognition. The need to be heard was vital. Along with any health care needs, that person's value was being undermined in her own eyes, and it represented a situation where emotional and spiritual support was necessary.

DECIDING TOGETHER

Sometimes families respond to the advice the doctors give them. This may be a knee jerk response, and in acting precipitously they can be in danger of infantilising their relative. Certainly, in this above case the patient did not fully understand, and saw it as a conspiracy that was threatening to take away her freedom and independence without her permission. Rarely is a change of circumstances such as I have described handled to the satisfaction of all parties. The main problem is that independence is the last bastion to fall before a person capitulates to the inevitable. No wonder people hang on to it tenaciously, even if they are too frail, forgetful or able to manage living on their own any more. It is rather tragic, but it is a fact of life.

Ideally, this decision should be one that the elderly person needs to come to themselves. Sometimes they do. Even with feelings of reluctance they will embrace the future having weighed up all the relevant information. They have come to accept the inevitable. I have seen it many times and try to affirm the wisdom and the pain of this move once it has been carefully assessed. Because losing our home is traumatic, it can feel like a portent about an uncertain future. The patient may well feel as if the reward for a lifetime of caring for others is that of being bundled off to a home for the convenience of others, even if this is far from the truth. I have an elderly mother who is fiercely independent, and all I can do is to advise with caution when asked. I cannot say that all her recent decisions for own independent status have been wise, but respect dictates that we allow people the dignity of their own decisions if they are able to make them. At some point in their lives they had to do that with us when we were their responsibility!

I always try to ask people how they feel about going into a residential home. Some react as if they have been cheated out of further years in a familiar environment. Others will admit that it had all been getting a bit much for them, and although they love their home, it is time to rationalise their life. The last approach is often the path of deeper peace.

The chief requirement in being aware of the post-fall possibilities is sensitivity. The need for people in a life transition involves being valued, finding meaning, having hope and having dignity, all factors present in any Spiritual Needs Assessment. We need to listen to people's feelings, but counsel caution in the interests of health and safety when it is clear that person is too weak to go back to the life they led before a fall. Elderly people are vulnerable persons. They may have been brought up not to acknowledge this term, but in today's relatively unsafe world it is actually the case. In the past families were less mobile, life expectancy was lower and communities as well as families gathered round those failing in their strength. Perhaps it is that closure is a necessity for some. This is by no means easy when their home may be the place where they lived with their partner, raised their children and was their base for as long as they remember. It may abound with many precious memories, happy and sad. It is a real bereavement, and perhaps that factor, often unacknowledged, that adds to the 'irrational' holding on with many elderly to being in their own home. We need to be tuned to these issues, even if people pass swiftly through our wards, and we may see them very little.

ADJUSTMENT - A WAY OF LIFE

In so many other ways it isn't just about falls. Illness and accident carry wide ranging consequences. I have looked into some of the adjustments for people with spinal and brain injuries. In their case the fact is that their lives can be altered radically. Others with different challenges experience this as well. An example might be someone with a kidney condition who may have to visit a hospital twice a week for lengthy dialysis. Those living with cancer may need chemotherapy or blood transfusions on a regular basis. All of these things make it less easy to live a "normal" life. People will have to adjust their sights to hope for less in life. They make need to make sacrifices. The daily or weekly routine will have to change to accommodate medical treatments, in the same way that others have to organise their week around the trip to the supermarket or hairdresser. From the situations I have encountered, I have found that people are enormously resilient in the face of these obstacles to a full life, and creative in their ways

103

of managing their disability. It can be humbling what people take on board without complaint, but that does not stop us learning to get the feel of what it might be like to them. It is no easy task for them. They deserve our understanding. We do not walk in their shoes.

Those who do draw alongside people experiencing the 'ripples in the pool' will possibly find themselves in admiration of the attitudes they witness. They might be fooled into believing that there is not a down side to conditions and treatments. There are huge losses that are probably also registering under the surface that accompany a downturn in health. I believe that exposure to people like this actually educates us to the wide range of responses to disappointment and difficult life adjustment that quietly go on 'out there'. I believe that they also show us that the resourcefulness of people under stress can in some instances be little short of amazing. Perhaps this cautions us to hold back from good advice to people in the management of their lifestyle changes unless we are specifically asked. Often affirming their own decisions gives them the confidence they require more than the "if I were you I would do this" approach that we can all fall into when we are not careful. After all is they who live with their challenges.

It is inevitably painful to us when we encounter people whose lives appear to us to be diminishing and it will probably affect us emotionally. We may be tempted to try and 'rescue' them. As I heard recently at a Palliative Care conference in the Royal Marsden Hospital, "it does not cost more to be compassionate, but it *is* more draining." The reality is that we might be in the same boat in the future, none of us knows. What is known is that we are fellow travellers with them. Our task is to affirm them as they develop their life skills according to who they are, which may be more a question of giving them back the power that their health may have denied them as they carry on their journey. All this is good spiritual care; quality care.

20

THE TRAUMA OF SHATTERED DREAMS

We like the world around us which we inhabit to be the shape we want it to be. That is understandable; we all tend to be like that. However, putting this differently, we like a permanent comfort zone, where everything is predictable and works out for our good. We learn over the years to realise that it just is not like that.

Popular ideas about our life prospects, success on several fronts and a hope for the future, generally omit the possibility of ill-health, serious or otherwise. Sudden illness and deeply offend our sense of order. They challenge our philosophy of how life should be. Our plans for the next few years rarely take illness into account, unless it is an elective operation like a hip replacement. Most people who find themselves in hospital unexpectedly, may have stepped onto the street that day without thinking that they would meet with an accident. Of course we don't think like that, but it is worth bearing in mind that it is not morbid and it would do no harm to risk assess when appropriate. The older we get the more likely we are to wake up to the fact that thinking twice before we do something can yield rewards. At the simplest level, it is wise to take note of the weather forecast before you go out and take the appropriate wear for the conditions.

Popular or conventional wisdom has much to be responsible for in its denial of the dark side of life. Even if we don't have a particular faith or a recognising of a higher power, just doing all the 'right' things does not render us immune from illness and misadventure. Patients in hospital often go through life changing experiences that make them think differently in the future, and it often causes them to re-evaluate their priorities and life values.

Every culture will have certain ways of enshrining popular or conventional wisdom. These may be found in sacred writings or in throwaway lines heard in television 'soaps'. We've imbibed them from our earliest years from all manner of sources; home and family, relatives, schools and the institutions we may have attended. What might they sound like? They vary, but certainly in the culture in which I was brought up they often sound like this:

> What goes around comes around.
> Work hard and you'll succeed.
> Do (or believe) X, Y and Z and you'll go to heaven.
> People get what they deserve.
> Keep your nose clean and you'll get by.
> You reap what you sow.
> Take regular exercise, eat plenty of greens and you'll be fit and happy.
> If you are good you will live long, have good health and prosper.
> When the going gets tough, the tough get going.

Whilst we may internalise these and other similar catch phrases, many of us are unconsciously committed to a performance and rewards view of life. If we do the right thing we will be rewarded. Deep down we think that quality of our life depends on doing things right. Perhaps this goes some of the way to explaining the shock reactions to illness, accident and disability that we find 'when the balloon goes up.'

To try to illustrate this, as part of Staff Induction in hospital we would talk about how we look on life when all is going well. How generally we can be optimistic in our worldview. We know, of course that bad things including ill health and accident happen to people, but somehow it will not happen to us. If it does, theoretically speaking, we think that we will manage the experience with good grace and some fortitude. To illustrate this we blow up a balloon, saying, as people started to look worried, fearing the balloon might burst noisily, "this how we might sum up our received worldview and the conventional wisdom that fills it." But when the crisis does occur, rather than the balloon holding up, it deflates. Inside we often resemble that deflated balloon. It represents the dismay at being let down by our philosophy of life. A deflated balloon looks rather wretched, shrivelled and floppy. This demonstration tended to make the point quite effectively.

An inflated balloon can represent our view of the world and is part of the unconscious understanding we hold of the way the world is. These concepts are learned from the womb and reinforced in our families and social circles and rarely questioned. They are assumed and are rarely questioned until the balloon metaphorically goes up! These concepts will cover things like what happens to us in life and how we might respond to it. This can often be blindly optimistic. However, as many people discover, the 'balloon of hope' may deflate rather alarmingly or even burst when the world treats you badly. Healthcare personnel need to treasure the development of sensitivity to respond to people's shattered dreams. They represent loss. Hospitals can be graveyards of discarded ambitions. In the same way, our internal experience at that time might be likened to the jigsaw puzzle that falls onto the floor. The pieces may all still be there, but somehow it is almost imposssible to assemble quickly enough them into a coherent picture. This can make people despair. It is a metaphor for the fragmentation illness and trauma can bring about in a sensitive person. "I am all over the place", is a statement that conveys this inner position. It is hard in a fragmented state of mind, to put the picture back together without sensitive help and support.

THE NEED FOR BEING IN CHARGE

It is no wonder then that people just like us who experience an event or experience which is not expected from the picture presented to us by conventional wisdom or popular culture may fragment inside. "I don't know what is going on!" or "I can't understand why this is happening to me" may be widespread reactions. The contemporary myth of infallibility tends to promote a false sense of indestructibility within us, as well as the inaccurate notion that we can control everything around us. People are shocked when their bodies let them down. When we cry out in our pain, "why me?" it is a perfectly understandable reaction to sudden stress. However, how often do you hear people asking '"why them?" The usual occasion you hear this is when bad things happen to those that we imagine are the kinds of people who are immune to disaster within the terms of conventional wisdom. This may include celebrities, very wealthy people and perhaps saintly people. The contemporary and descriptive term "shit happens" may not fall comfortably upon our ears but it certainly sums up the reality of life. Illness, accident and even death are no respecter of persons. Pariahs of society such as hit and run drivers, illegal immigrants, substance abusers as well as duchesses, judges and popular celebrities are all likely to get ill at some point in their lives. Today's Celeb culture paints a rosy picture of the impossible which is seductive and unhelpful. It breeds dissatisfaction with what we have. We want the high life, and we want it to come easy. Life can be very tough. Even celebs have skeletons in their cupboards as recent Jimmy Savile revelations have brought to light.

The media contain stories of sudden or premature accident or death all the time. It is not all 'out there', remote from us all. It can come dangerously close. While some lifestyle choices will increase the likelihood for some, it does not mean that the others will be somehow bypassed in this respect.

LIFESTYLE AND LIABILITY

We are very health conscious today. We have been buttonholed in our present generation by advertising which invites a growing dependence on diets and vitamins, gyms and health spas or more extreme practices such as colonic irrigation. The lure of perfect physical and mental fitness whispers to us from every angle. Cosmetic surgery allows the wealthy to choose the kind of physical attributes they want. Celebrity magazines can encourage us down this road. It all panders to our insecurity and desire to be loved and esteemed.

Health and lifestyle have become education issues today. The government is worried about obesity; smoking has been banished outdoors, and drinking on a huge scale is worrying politicians and the health organisations greatly. Celebrity endorsements of diets and techniques act to further bolster our belief of their efficacy. Food and exercise regimes, alternative therapies and in vogue or endorsed diets attract a following. There are few magic answers in life! Many health promotion strategies may actually be beneficial, although we may need to do our homework on them. The same suggestion of achievable immortality that is present in conventional wisdom is also present in this climate of a preoccupation with primary health. It is no bad thing, though I suspect it appeals to our insecurities, and the promoters of most products have a strong financial agenda. The myth remains however, if you jettison junk food, run marathons or eat plenty of broccoli you will take off weight, become very fit and stave off cancer. But is this the whole truth?

I have listened to many people in hospital telling me that they were fit, took exercise and watched their diet and how they cannot understand how they are now facing a prostate procedure or heart surgery. I can understand their surprise, but fit people still have physical problems that catch them unawares. I contracted viral pneumonia the day after doing some intensive training in a local park. We are no different to a motor vehicle in this respect. When your car does not start one morning, the likelihood is that you will have driven it quite satisfactorily to your home the evening before. That has happened to me several times. When you ask the mechanic about it, all they usually tell you is that this or that has gone and it needs replacing or mending. Is some ways the human body is similar. By the same token, the higher the mileage or older the vehicle, the more likely it is to break down!

At the same time as our health and fitness concerns us we seem also find obesity to be a worrying problem for others. In the last decades it has been noted by Government that as a population we have become more obese, less fit and more prone to all kinds of lifestyle diseases than ever. The reality is that over the last sixty years, the rise of technology has provided us with more and more labour saving devices, and the standard of living linked to the ability to defer payment has enabled us to purchase them. Advertisements coming from all sides can lure us into buying the latest thing and not doing so may lead to the threat of social exclusion. When we do not have the latest gadgetry we don't usually die. The Joneses need a lot of keeping up with! The cult of celebrity can be a toxic mirage that can affect our psychological health and our pockets. Technology today can be subtly conspiratorial, and we find ourselves colluding passively with planned obsolescence. Before long we are *have* to 'update' our devices. That costs money; and if we have not got it, it increases stress which we need even less than the latest 'must-have' gadget.

A further possibility in today's world is the lure of cosmetic surgery without sound medical reason and the pursuit of the body beautiful, unheard of when the NHS began. Here the celebrity lure may strike again! These things play on our human insecurities and are also insidious agents of mounting financial pressure, creating stresses that are really not good for health. Research over in the past decade has linked stress to heart disease **(43)** chronic fatigue **(44)** and the fact that it hinders the healing process **(45)** and ages the immune system. **(46)**

BASIC FITNESS

Further influences on our present state of health and fitness may have arisen through sociological and practical changes in the home. Home has often been where women have in the past experienced a kind of domestic slavery. Nowadays we see a change in patterns of employment whereby women have jobs away from the home. These factors allied to increased technology have provided other reasons to adopt labour saving devices like dishwashers, washing machines, and for the garden such devices as leaf blowing machines and garden strimmers. In the past we made our own bread, washed our own clothes and cleaned houses the laborious way. The domestic workload and lower standard of living - no fast food and instant meals out - ensured a different kind of physical fitness. Washing machines, vacuum cleaners and even dishwashers are now seen as necessary fixtures. Heavy industry like mining that once developed great physical strength, particularly in men along with manual work in the factory and on the land has diminished. Public and private transport has made us less inclined to walk very much anymore.

This is all a very different world to the one in which the concept of the National Health Service was conceived. Even the social changes typified by high mobility, a pluralist society with wide choice lead to stress, uncertainty and an underlying pressure to keep pace with the current trends. We work long hours, we play hard, we can reach for the moon in many ways, and yet some of the basic human ills remain. Easy access to drugs and alcohol has been responsible for many hospital admissions over the years, not least on a Friday and Saturday night in Accident and Emergency departments. Poverty still remains a big problem, not least among children while domestic abuse and violence are still around. All of this puts pressure on the Health Service. In fact the grounds for conventional wisdom of the kind that I have described are not justified by the evidence that faces us every day. Unless of course we live in an ivory tower, and few can afford *them*!

What do we do when the promises of perfect health don't deliver? As responsible and thinking adults we all have to find our own way through life. We also possess our own forms of wisdom or makeshift security blankets. Sometimes they work for us, sometimes we may have to admit they don't. What we can helpfully do for people when they don't, is to listen to and accept their dismay at being let down. This betrayal is hard to take, whether by their bodies, God, their value system or indeed the wisdom inherited from early years in an uncritical way. It is a kindness to allow people their own feelings when the pain of disappointment hits them and not try to reason with them. Life, we have to recognise, is cruel sometimes, and the disappointment that people feel is very real. *Sometimes the answer is that there are no answers.* That should not stop anybody asking the serious questions that arise from a feeling of betrayal. In my experience people come to terms with difficult events, particularly in relation to health issues if we let them do the questioning and let them come to their own conclusions. To do this is a measure of the holistic and spiritual care that may be called upon many times a day in the hospital setting, where so many of these issues have a habit of surfacing. Sickness, accident and disability can be cruel and can so easily alter the shape we hope the world will be. Is this a trauma; in subtle ways, I believe so.

21

THE WISDOM TO LISTEN

"If we could all just learn to listen, everything else would fall into place. Listening is the key to being patient- centred" (47) In saying this Ian Mcwhinney (who has been called ' the Father of Family Medicine') records his reflection on many decades of G.P. practice.

Being present to people is sometimes all that is required by a person undergoing crisis. People don't always want answers. When in shock, the present for them is a very foggy business. Readymade answers are not wanted or sought even if people are asking "why?" In his 2008 paper on Compassion in Healthcare, Robin Youngson observes: "There is compelling research from the Studer Group to show that empathetic concern and investing time up front to check a patient's needs increases efficiency and patient satisfaction. An hourly round of patients by nurses dramatically of call buttons, freeing up nursing time."(48)

When people are feeling vulnerable, disorientated and not 'at home' in health care surroundings, one of the simplest healing approaches is that of focused and interested listening to people. This can often contain a person's feelings, making them feel both understood and safe. Sometimes it is just 'being there' and staying with the pain of the situation that can be more effective than the most heroic gesture. As the actor and director, Woody Allen has been quoted as saying, "95% of life is just about showing up." This facility of 'being there' we discover is an art more than a science.

When people have lost a loved one and are bereaved, they often enter a dark valley. They can often feel are isolated. They find that they cannot reach out beyond their grief, and no one can enter their world. That does not mean we stay away. On the contrary, more comfort than we realise is brought by people who have the courage to continue their relationship with the bereaved person but in a quiet way, and with their permission. Just being there, another 'body around the place' can bring more gentle healing to the wounded than we think. Making 'a cuppa' can convey more than a lecture on survival after bereavement.

WORDS WITHOUT WORDS

Superficial politeness is trained into many people from an early age. An example of this is when someone asks you, "how are you?" and we reply "fine, thank you," when perhaps that is not entirely true. Once, when being very mischievous a few years ago, I thought I would test this one out. Someone I knew asked me the same question and I replied "suicidal". They continued as if I had said "fine"! That person might not pass muster as a patient visitor. Listening attentively is very important. By doing so we can differentiate between a person saying that they are well with their lips and the manner in which they say it The latter may lend the lie to their affirmations of total wellbeing. In fact my colleagues are well used to being told than people in hospital beds are fine. Inevitably the unvoiced question comes immediately to mind "then why are you in hospital?" Of course this somewhat 'british' approach is largely a defence mechanism to avoid the loss of equilibrium. To many this response will seem less than wise because reality is more of a friend long term than unreality, especially when you are ill.

A lack of appropriate attentiveness can be found anywhere; sadly in the caring professions too. A colleague one told me of a particular visit he made to his G.P. As he entered the consulting room, the doctor was glued to the monitor in front of him. He did not even look up as he ushered my friend into a chair with a sweep of the hand. He proceeded to ask the screen what the trouble was. My friend considered this very poor practice. Good listening is about holding eye contact, having an open stance, and showing them value by a sense of our polite interest. Good listening is also about bracketing our *own* feelings and issues so that they do not invade the present encounter in any way. Good listening is also about reflecting back what the person is saying in order that they know that *you* have heard, and that helps them hear, perhaps for the first time, what they are expressing to you! A revelation may occur.

PICKING UP SIGNALS

In listening actively to people I would say it is not our job either to suggest that they are not telling truth nor is it our job to attempt to psychoanalyse them. What we do in fact is to discern from people's words and body language the emotional place where they are coming from. We cannot not be successful in doing this with everyone, possibly no one is. It is an awareness to be learned. However by listening with the whole of ourselves to the whole of that other person we learn much more about their interior world, the one that matters, than the surface only. In Family Therapy, there is a phrase that sums this up perfectly, and it is *we cannot **not** communicate*. What this suggests is that we unconsciously communicate all sorts of things about ourselves, our hopes and fears and anxieties just by the manner in which we speak and how we deport ourselves. Only we don't know it, but our listener may!

The Chinese pictogram for 'to listen', at first glance looks like a series of squiggles. In fact this character sums up much of what any counselling course would include within the art of listening. In this character you have an ear shape shown because primarily we listen with our ears. To this is added the part of the character that expresses 'you' because it is *you* who listens to another person. Below this shape are the three eyes, the two physical eyes we possess and the inner eye, the eye of our perception. Beneath the eyes is an unbroken line that denotes undivided attention, and below that is a depiction of the heart, because we listen to people with our hearts open to them. I think this expresses a deep truth and is a wonderful and concise picture. I personally find it such a helpful approach to listening skills, and it demonstrates that ancient cultures had a deep understanding of the place of listening in human support and comfort. It may not be first nature to ourselves, so that we often have to work hard to emulate it.

UNCONDITIONAL POSITIVE REGARD

The writer and therapist Dr Carl Rogers coined an expression that conveyed the attitude of the listener to the client. He called it "unconditional positive regard" (**49**) but in essence it is about affirming the story and signals flowing from the listener by being interested and warmly accepting of all that he or she is being told unconditionally.

I can think of many, many instances where the use of our eyes has communicated acceptance, and something like "I am here for you." Over a period of several decades, I have encountered people of all backgrounds, genders and experience of life who have broken down in tears at a look, a gesture or some gentle introductory words. A colleague of mind simply asked a junior doctor how they were and they burst into floods of tears. This young doctor was very tired and felt that they were responsible for a very bad mistake recently in the course of their practice. This simple enquiry opened the floodgates and they were able to explore together the truth of the matter, which in fact was not as terrible as that doctor's perception of it. I was walking down a street in London once when I saw someone I knew quite well. As I engaged their eyes they just fell into uncontrollable sobs. Clearly they had a bad day, but it was the sight of a friend that brought out the grief.

In hospital this kind of entering the 'holy of holies' of people's inner lives is truly a privilege. To avoid the risk of being 'fools who rush in' we really do need to give some serious attention to the art of listening.

Having been through some challenging experiences with my own family over the years, I have often been amazed at how our own life experience, our downs probably more than our ups, can feed the lives of others. This happens in reverse, of course. A week after some anxious moments as a parent, I found myself listening to two people on the same day, one a staff member and also a patient about their health which had been affected by relationships. It helps to identify with situations that people describe. As I listened I found personal bells ringing with the stories that both these people had to tell. Whilst the majority of the time spent in each of these engagements was spent listening, I found myself mirroring back very similar things to each of them. There was a connection. I think it was probably because I had 'been there', and our encounters were about being in the right place at the right time. It struck me then that it is our relationships with people that bring about our deepest joys and our greatest agonies in life. In other words, as the phrase goes, nobody on their death bed says, "I wish I had spent more time in the office."

FACILITATING HEALTHY CHOICE

Both people these people I encountered had health issues that they were presenting with. Not very long into the conversation the issue of unreliable boyfriends arose. I found as I was listening that these people actually needed a third party with whom they could bounce off some of their ideas and queries and mental wrestling. There were decisions to make within their very different situations. They were both effectively saying "I don't think this relationship is doing me any good. My health is suffering and at the centre of it all is how I feel about the way they treat me." It was not my job to collude, but I could certainly understand and affirm their thought processes. From my own life experiences I could see patterns and principles emerging that tend to govern the success or otherwise of a lot of relationships. I often feel each of us knows more than we admit to ourselves about what we should do in situations. Mostly we resist facing loss. We want others to support us, not by applying pressure, but simply by listening and helping them through the issues by reflecting back what they are saying so they can hear themselves, perhaps for the first time.

One person I met was trying to deal with the stranglehold of a drink and drugs problem, that her boyfriend was only making worse. Her decision in leaving hospital was whether to live with her sister for a while, which would have given her time, space and support to get better. However this would have put her boyfriend out. The alternative course of action for her would be to return to his flat where his friends would be dropping by to encourage habits from which she was trying to break free. In modern parlance that would be a 'no brainer'; but when emotions and the dynamics of relationships are involved, it was no easy matter. I could have said what I felt, but that would be imposing my view. All I could do was to reflect back to her the path she was hesitantly embarking on. I just hoped she made the right decision for her to learn from the wake- up call of her illness. In listening we have to let people go, and avoid the temptation to get over

116

involved in situations that are not ours to solve. It can be painful, but it can leave people free to grow in their own way.

SHARING THE DARKNESS

We cannot truly enter the difficult world of another without also feeling some of the suffocating atmosphere of a life diminishing. In listening there is little to be gained in the proverbial shouting loudly from the top of the slimy pit, "Hey, it's great up here, you should come up and see for yourself!" If a person could they would! It is little short of insulting to speak from the world of the fit and able to the restricted world of the weak and powerless. Emotionally we make better contact if we were to metaphorically enter the slimy pit alongside them as best as we can, to close the gap and make the dark place inhabitable for the other by sharing a little of the experience.

Henri Nouwen puts it in this way: "Those who do not run away from our pains but touch them with compassion bring healing and new strength. The paradox indeed is that the beginning of healing is the solidarity with the pain. In our solution-based society it is more important than ever to realise that wanting to alleviate pain without sharing it is like wanting to save a child from a burning house without the risk of being hurt." **(50)**

22

Touch; an agent of healing

"Thank you . . ."
"Sorry?"
Thank you for touching me . . ."
"Oh, but surely lots of people touch you . . ."
"No, a lot of people handle me. You touched me . . . thank you."

This incident describes how a volunteer visitor was once thanked profusely for touching a patient gently on the shoulder. When questioned, the patient said that although many people did in fact handle her over the course of the day, a *meaningful* touch meant so much more. The sensitive and non-invasive touch, look, or gentle enquiry often adds a significant affirmative sense of regard for people who might otherwise feel they are the property of the hospital and not people at all.

It is all part of the experience of being unwell and in hospital that people can become isolated. Pain isolates people because the only person who can feel that pain is the patient themselves. Saying things like "I know how you feel" is really little help at all because it is unlikely that anyone bar the patient themselves can feel that specific pain. Taking pain seriously is not an easy thing to do. Sometimes pain is the only thing that a person can deal with at one time. Even close friendships have to take second place to pain.

A light touch however can sometimes break the isolation. I am quite tactile, but chaplains are cautioned in their training of the dangers of an over familiar attitude when we are with patients. I think again you need to discern who you are with, but a little gentle touch on the shoulder or elbow is a non- verbal sign of solidarity and reassurance. On the occasions when I am asked to pray with people, they will invariably give me their hand as I do so. It is a precious moment of connection.

Communication levels are so important to people who feel that they may be drifting away from the mainstream of living. A look that tells someone that you can *see* can speak volumes. Somehow effective communications like listening and the touch that lets people know that they are a precious human being are art forms to be learned. The learning comes slowly and often through experience. As David Stoter, former Head of Chaplaincy at the Queen's Medical Centre in Nottingham tells us, "Communication skills involve a great deal more than simply talking to a person and passing on information." **(51)**

As the majority of professionals who interact with a patient in hospital are either *after* something like blood or basic observation information, someone who is interested in you personally can be quite pleasing and surprising. Other more clinical staff may sometimes see you as "the appendix" and bypass your personhood in getting to the root of the physical problem. This is all well and good, except that once a person becomes vulnerable because they may feel they are helplessly drifting away from the shores of ordinary human interaction, they will want more felt recognition of who are they are. People have stories. Our own story has led us to the point at which a specialist or a nurse meets and interacts with us. Little things can mean a lot, even a touch.

My observation over the years is that domestic staff can often restore a person's sense of self by the simple remembering of their name or how many sugars they take in their tea. One day I was surprised to encounter a cleaner on a Neuro-Physiological ward waltzing a patient round the space between the rows of beds! A maverick approach, perhaps, but from what I observed somehow that action brought a precious piece of humanity back to a place and a person where it had been previously ebbing away.

The manner of communication does not always have to be verbal. To experience good communication is a spiritual need, however it works out. Beth Perry says; "Entranced by your eyes, the messages come strongly and swiftly. As you reach out to me, you complete the circuit. For a moment we are one, understanding each other completely." **(52)** In this way the conveyance of essential humanity across the space between patient and healthcare staff is being described. To reiterate the maxim that we cannot *not* communicate- *everything* we do may be interpreted. In other words our body language can easily speak volumes to a patient where words fail.

It is a bit like the person who says "fine" when you ask how they are, but the words spoken are lent the lie by that discernible set of the jaw. This gives the game away. They are not fine at all, but they probably don't want to discuss it. They are making a communication, but not in the way they intended. It can be wise to move on. When this does occur, it's better not to challenge. The patient sets the agenda after all!

As health professionals or visitors entering a patient's world, we too will communicate things. How often a patient has spotted tiredness, distractedness or discomfort of some kind in me. I used to deny what they had observed, but learned that the gap bridged by honesty simply brings patient and professional closer. I think in our ignorance, we think we are always meant to be 'on top'. Who is, all the time?

THE NON- VERBAL: A HEALING COMMUNICATION

In 2001 a newspaper article described how two children of Nigel (a prominent rugby player and BBC rugby and Olympics commentator) and Ros Starmer-Smith contracted serious terminal illnesses within nine years. This was a huge blow in itself and one cannot imagine what the family went through during this time losing both Charlotte and Julian. These young people showed immense courage along with the family, in their combating of these illnesses. The staff at the John Radcliffe Hospital had also been very affected by this double tragedy. The specialist in charge of Julian said to the family "We have been learning things as well as you." The thing that really struck the staff was that they had seen love in its most naked state and this had struck home.

Julian's older brother Charles, who had a very good relationship with Julian would always have the right 'touch' in his support of Julian. At one point Julian's head was shaved because the chemotherapy was causing his hair to drop out. The treatment also meant he could not talk. In spite of this Charles and Julian did have beautiful communication. Without telling his family, Charles had his hair shaved. he came to his brother's bedside. Julian rubbed Charles's bald head and gave a thumbs up. It was the most intimate expression of what they meant to each other.

When he had a fever Charles seemed to know the way to calm Julian, who was thrashing around wildly, kicking out and gesticulating. Charles was the only person who Julian would respond to and Charles just held him hour after hour. He hugged him, lay with him on the bed and just calmed him down." As Nigel remarked, "It was just the most extraordinary depth of love I have ever seen." **(53)**

Clearly NHS staff are not always in a position to be doing this for their patients, but loved ones can. The point of describing this harrowing yet touching incident is to show that that the right touch given by the right person in the right way may be healing at its deepest level.

SEPARATION AT A STROKE

Over the years I have spent many hours with stroke patients. Among many of the effects of a stroke is loss of speech. This comes as a cruel blow at a point when people desperately want to explore what is happening to them. It isolates people even further. Not only have they had the shock of a stroke which usually comes unannounced, but if they cannot speak or articulate their thoughts and feelings, they become doubly isolated. I try to tell people that things often do improve. I found that I could not easily understand them when they had aphasia (affected speech).

Sometimes they lost all power of speech. It was not always easy to understand what they are trying to communicate. I learned to accept that was kinder to say that I did not catch what they were saying. I needed to do it in such a way as not to imply that it is was their fault. Again here touch could be powerful. I have known those who were left with only have one word like "yes" or "no" with which they answer every question. This may seem confusing. Actually the tone and emphasis seems to get across what they mean. One particular man only had the phrase "today's the day" which he used as a means of saying everything! He seemed happy with it, even if I was a bit lost at times. It is all still communication - of a kind!

As often as not I have found that the person's eyes and general facial expression will communicate enough of that person's interior world and feelings. That may give us a place to start. Stroke patients suffering from aphasia often can't get the right word out if they can speak. I sometimes ask them as they struggle to find the right word whether it might feel like going to a library shelf, intent of picking a specific title. When they take the chosen title, like the word they are searching for, down from the metaphorical shelf, it is not the title they wanted. It can be frustrating but in the patient's mind though that 'mis-word' seems to do.

I remember a woman I regularly visited years at home ago who had a stroke. While she was recovering, there was one occasion when she described the vicar as "the radiator", and also wished me a "happy conception" when she heard my wife and I were expecting our first child! Thankfully I knew what she meant. This woman also had a strange cat, which jumped into the base of a grandfather clock and hid whenever visitors came. It made me wonder whether the cat was not coping with its owner's strange stroke- induced Malapropisms, and hid to avoid embarrassment!

However when this strange speech glitch happens, it is almost something that is made harder by trying, like when we try to remember something on the tip of our tongue. The more you try the more the word escapes you. On many occasions swearing came more easily than a word or sentence that a person was struggling to get out. The swearing did actually express the frustration they felt very accurately. Not pretty but effective. It is though, necessary to try to engage in the disconnected world of the stroke patient and often it comforts them that you are prepared to make the effort.

BRIDGING THE GAP

It is worth saying that two people together can always make *some* kind of communication. Even those who for various reasons can only manage a grunt, can accompany this with a look or mannerism that is a clue to the general area of communication. The will to break the impasse that some medical conditions can bring about is a very important factor in the pastoral and spiritual care of people in hospital. That too, is where meaningful touch can speak as well.

People with tracheotomies and those who have to wear oxygen masks are impaired as well. Both make speech difficult and further isolate the patient. Alongside the isolation of illness for them comes the inability to communicate with another at a satisfactory level. Eye contact and appropriate touch, in spite of the frustration of not being able to carry on a satisfactory two way conversation, can break the social isolation. That kind of touch may be affirming and personal without being unnecessarily intimate. It may communicate that sense of "I wish I could do more" or "hang in there". It may bridge the space between that person and yourself in a way words perhaps cannot.

All this is about social isolation caused by illness, particularly strokes, and what we can do to lessen the gap. Another human being at 'the other end of the line' is very reassuring to people, even if that human being, if they are anything like me, feel as if they are floundering a lot of the time. Helplessness, as we shall see in a later chapter can often be a prerequisite for staying with the vulnerable. The experience of floundering may actually no obstacle to closing the distance on that person's sense of isolation. This sense of powerlessness may be in itself a meaningful sacrifice to our desired wish for competency, rather than a failure, a perception that we often need a lot of persuading to embrace. We like to be in control!

23

THE VALUED BALM OF COMPASSION AND COMPANIONSHIP

"Compassion is an assumed value but it is scarcely mentioned in any of the documents about healthcare strategies or aspirations. When I searched the websites of all the quality-improvement organisations I was unable to find the word 'compassion' at all." (54) So Robin Youngson noticed from his New Zealand experience. Perhaps when we look at the roots of the words *care, compassion* and *companion* what we get is a sense of engagement, not detachment. I believe this is a perennial challenge for any health service, when time and resources compete with the humanitarian agenda.

As with my experience of tonsillectomy as a boy, the fact that others were going through the same roller coaster of buffets, rigours and anxieties was a comfort, thus the reason why victims of major incidents are often grouped together in the same ward. The companionship of shared events, however traumatic, can offer a balm for healing to that series of happenings, as shocking as they were in the early days. Fellow travellers around you seem to reinforce the message that 'somebody understands'. This is sound wisdom in the hospital's response to a major incident. I saw this at first hand after the Great Heck train crash of 2001. I did a lot of visiting at that time on one particular ward, but I sensed was an evident gulf between me and the survivors which no amount of empathy could bridge. They were pleased to communicate with me at length. What was better was to have a wounded and surviving person in the next bed. It was companionship at its best, and a healing balm to the inner wounds which would take much longer to heal.

In the preceding chapters I have tried to describe some of the patient experiences that accompanies the event of hospitalisation and ill health. I have touched upon the collateral damage experienced by the family and loved ones of the patient. From my own experience of working alongside countless people in hospital, I have been made aware that the NHS tends toward 'curing' rather than 'caring' when they use the term "care". They are not the same thing. The word 'care' comes from *kara* (Gothic) and means 'weeping'. These words actually denote a human response to others' suffering of deep involvement and not detachment. It costs to care. For many it is the accompanying experience of vulnerability, alienation and anxiety that causes as much concern as the diagnosis and treatment of the presenting physical condition. There are as many people who are deeply worried about how their dog is going to get along, or whether their home will stand up to the winter weather conditions as are worried about how the surgeons are going to deal with their gall bladder or hip replacement.

I have a feeling that the emotional experiences of the patient or the deeper needs of human spirit when encountering ill health are simply not included in the "care". Too often when a person is fragmenting emotionally under the worries they are feeling, a clinical psychiatrist (or even a chaplain) may be called for by staff. This can be very helpful and a desired intervention. Some people will feel they are being treated as being "different" and a little "strange" when a professional who specialises in the mental side of things, or wears a clerical collar is brought in. To my mind the rhetoric of holistic care that is often quoted in both NHS and hospital publications pays lip service to an ideal if the *total* condition of a person is not given equal weight to the purely physical. As Elisabeth Kubler-Ross has emphasised: "If we could combine the teaching of the new scientific and technical achievements with equal emphasis on interpersonal human relationships we would indeed make progress, but not if the new knowledge is conveyed to the student at the price of less and less interpersonal contact". (55)

Yet for the past fourteen years I have spent hours with people who have just been given bad news or are bewildered by the communication given by the doctors about the treatment they are being given. This raises the whole issue regarding a diminishing of the human spirit which has not been seen as part and parcel of being admitted to hospital. It just has to be seen as low level trauma. To my mind these inner, deeper elements too, touch on the broader aspects of health. It is a *person* who is frightened, frustrated or confused. The body does not thrive if anxieties are rampant as they are regularly when our health breaks down. We will need a certain level of stress free space to recover. The World Health Organisation certainly believes these things to be fundamental in their definition of health.

Clearly the need for support is present. How might it be achieved? The first thing that strikes me is that in the pressured environment of the hospital ward, time is at a premium. Many hospital staff often end up appearing to be somewhat manic. It cannot really be helped. Unfortunately the quality of care suffers. It's a fact of life. When a person wants a bed pan or is chivvying up a nurse for a pain killer promised half an hour previously, the response is often "in a minute". All too often the minute becomes an hour. Many feel bad about continuing to ask. They don't like to be a nuisance.

Open ended time is a precious commodity on the wards. Often the most helpful part of the body to a desperate patient is another's impartial, non-judgmental ear. The nurse who listened to me over thirty years ago had the luxury of time. It is no longer there. Things have changed immeasurably over the years. Today personnel such as volunteers, visitors, therapists, chaplains, domestic staff and porters often do have the time. Their role is invaluable in given the patient back their sense of being a human being as well as a patient. It is clear that many people within the hospital setting, if their heart is in the right place, can do the job of empathetic, compassionate and sensitive patient support. I think of our chaplaincy volunteers who do this job very well. Many doctors, nurses and therapists as well as porters and domestic staff do it with great effect. The point is made that the wider brief of holistic and spiritual care does not have to be the domain of "professionals" alone. Those with awareness, sensitivity and compassion are as vital to health as the highly trained medical practitioners. One of their greatest assets of the non-professional is the time to accompany the anxious in that place of uncertainty.

SOMETHING WE CAN *ALL* DO

"Thank you for listening" is often a phrase I hear when doing ward visits. Sometimes that is all that is required. Chapter 21 addresses this area at greater depth. People do not want bright ideas or "if I were you" statements or indeed shock reactions to what they are saying. There is nothing so containing to the vulnerable individual as the warm and accepting response of the listener who is able to convey understanding and concern. Sometimes words are not even necessary. It is probably this sense of companionship on the journey that most people will be wanting. People often value someone, even a stranger, willing to hear the pain behind the words, or the anxiety masked by the cheery face without making a fuss.

Listening is offering the hospitality of the heart. It breathes acceptance to the cautious discloser of information that may feel unacceptable. As Tuckwell and Flagg remind us, listening opens doors that maybe need that ventilation; "Yet, on listening, we may find that the root of real illness and pain is not in physical illness but rather in the emotional, psychological, social or spiritual experience of the individual."(56)

Just think for a moment on what hairdressers, taxi drivers, chiropodists and the like will hear in the course of a week, and how they find themselves acting as listeners when their purpose is primarily to either convey a person in their car or tend to their physical needs. So it is in hospital. Imagine what the therapists and dieticians hear. "I know what it's like" is probably much better expressed by an emotional bearing of a 'knowing' calm rather than spelling it out to a hurting person in words. We never know what it is like for others. They will know anyway by someone's manner whether they are being 'heard'. In any case, we only know what *we* have felt in a given circumstance. We will not know how another feels, only *they* will.

It's the same with physical pain. How often do people in hospital have to deal with a gnawing and nagging pain. How can people really have a feel for what *they* are enduring? It is not as if a person in pain can break off a piece and give it to another to experience. Only they have that particular - often indescribable - experience. Also different people have different pain thresholds. It is however, perfectly possible to say to someone clearly afflicted in this way," you must be in considerable pain. I cannot possibly imagine what you are going through, but I can see it in your face." This may not be an appropriate response for everyone, as some people are rightly very private about their pain, or indeed very angry. For some though that approach will certainly help them suddenly feel less isolated by that pain. Someone who understands that isolation becomes a companion.

COMPANIONS

The word *companion* comes to us via Middle English from the Old French which is based on Latin and means literally, "one who breaks bread with another". It is a noun of sharing. Again like the word *compassion* that also comes originally from the same root as companion, when broken into its component parts literally means "suffer with "; it denotes sharing at a deep level. (Incidentally the Latin verb *patior* from which the words patient and compassion come means 'to suffer' – an insight into both sickness and support in itself) Why have these words persisted in our language? I wonder perhaps whether it is because they describe a source of fellow feeling and healing presence that we human beings desperately need. People often say after a tragedy or humiliating experience, "You know who your real friends are." The likelihood is that they are the compassionate, caring and companionable ones. A compassionate companion must be like gold dust - dare I say manna in the desert - to the suffering person in hospital. We can convey this kind of solidarity just as well non-verbally. It is usually very much appreciated.

A classic example of the fusion between care, compassion and companionship comes in the parable of the Good Samaritan in Luke's Gospel, which I go into more lengths over in Chapter 29.

There is plenty of emotional and spiritual pain around in the healthcare setting. We have looked at spiritual pain and distress in Chapter 15. All pain will possess a spiritual aspect because the *meaning* of persons is begged by something as intolerable as physical (and emotional) pain. Accordingly as people will be asking the "why" questions about how they come to this place of helplessness. This has been my own experience. Marlene, who had recently heard bad news about cancer was very bewildered about why this was happening to her. "It doesn't seem right" she said to me.

128

Only too often the call-outs at night were to do with loss relating to both adult and babies. Imagine entering a room with the mother, sometimes partner and grandparents with that sense of emptiness and "why" resounding off the walls. A small motionless figure, draped in baby clothes and a bonnet, often a size too large, was a focal point in a family scene filled with tears and shock. I was then expected to bless that little baby. It was hard. One of my colleagues had to conduct around fifty neonatal and still birth funerals in one calendar year, and our Trust was no different to any other in this respect! Over these sad occasions, he just had to 'journey with' those grieving families.

There were many uncomfortable moments like attending to late miscarriages and baby deaths. It was particularly distressing when this was not the first for the family. There were times when I felt I was being seen as a magic figure who might just say those words which makes sense of the senseless. I couldn't, and often had to share in that moment of bewilderment and dereliction, with the "why" question hanging in the air. The issue of suffering that has no meaning has been addressed elsewhere, but it is certainly the hardest to accept. I am afraid there were not often clear answers as to why those babies died before they came to term. I simply had to enter that darkness with those people without the enlightening words.

When I was paged once onto Accident and Emergency to support a family shortly after the loss of a small child, run over whilst in a buggy on a shopping street, I felt thrown in at the deep end. I seriously wished I was not there in this stark hospital room full of people who are traumatised. Perhaps it was the obvious fact that I was a clergyman that seemed to mock the situation. "What kind of God would allow this?" was unspoken but present (like the proverbial elephant) in the room. As we have seen, a sense of powerless is often experienced in the face of deep and unwarranted suffering. I could only sit there amongst them and hope at some point that they would see I had no glib answers; but I *was there*.

Another issue that lay behind my appearance at a patient's bedside, whether at the end or as a referral by the ward or themselves is that of childhood abuse. Whether this be physical, sexual or emotional, the person was acutely aware that it had stayed with them as a predominant feature of their life. According to D.H. Lawrence "I am not a mechanism, an assembly of various parts. And it is not because the mechanism is working wrongly that I am ill. I am ill because of wounds to the soul, to the deep emotional self, and the wounds to the soul take a long long time, only time can help, and patience, and a certain difficult repentance" (**57**)

Sometimes one service I could offer was that of hearing people without judging and believing what they had to say. This simple intervention would often lead to a sense of more peace, like a confession made. Even on their deathbed, some needed to share this treatment that others had inflicted on them in order to "move on". I am not sure how much research backs this up, but abuse was a factor for some people who had been facing a lifetime of illness. This awful breakdown of trust and personal trauma seems to sap the life out of those who have been the victim of the negative attention of others. Certainly there is much research on the effect of stress in illness, and I cannot imagine a more persistent and undermining source of stress than abuse. A report of the House of Bishops entitled "A Time to heal "noted that "Emotional dis-ease lies behind many illnesses. The breakdown of relationship in marriages, families and other human groups strains the well-being of those involved. Drug addiction and alcoholism, the abuse of the human body and mind, and the prevalence of crime, violence and racism are signs of a deep rooted sickness in our local and national life." (**58**)

BEING THERE

In my years on the wards, in supporting those battling sickness and the experience of hospitalisation, I found often very little needed to be said. Being there is a first step. Perhaps others have made themselves absent because of the suffering of others, and it hurts. Understanding can come through a look, a touch, a gentle resigned nodding of the head. In those simple gestures the inner understanding you have gets through to the other and there is a meeting. "Thank you for listening" always seemed superfluous when that was primarily my role. Unlike some very keen Christians and militant atheists may assume, it is this gentler accompaniment of the sick and indisposed that was our priority rather than pushing religion at vulnerable patients. Interestingly enough some of my most memorable encounters were with self- confessed atheists. I was interested in them for who they were, and I think once we got over our mutual threat, we could be people together. However, when someone says that they valued your listening, you know you have touched a life, perhaps minimally, but at a time when it meant something. There were also times when longer conversations took place. In that situation it was a case of being at the right place at the right time. Often that time never came again; the moment passed. even the people who had shared from the depths of their being on one occasion seemed to have moved on when I next saw them, or they did not want to venture into that hurting, sensitive place again.

One of the saddest things we encounter is that very little of the support in being a compassionate companion for people in hospital requires much more than being a human being with some awareness and willingness to 'be there' when it matters. This seems sadly to be in short supply. Over the years our department received many 'thank you' letters. Many thank us for visiting on a daily basis. None of these letters suggested we did any more than stay with people in their bewilderment, pain or anxiety. These letters would variously describe "your kind and comforting support," "encouragement and companionship," "for being there", "your talks. . .kept me going," "for giving me the will to live," "love and support," and "kindness and caring." Little in these kinds of responses suggests great expertise was coming from us but they do express gratitude that when it was needed support came. It had helped to get people through a difficult time. Of all the people who have regular contact with patients how many could offer similar sensitive care? Yet when we ran courses for Staff Induction and spelt out the need for pastoral, spiritual and sometimes religious care, we often encountered threat, defensiveness, ignorance and the attitude of 'this isn't for us!' In one evaluation of the module (and it generally evaluated extremely well), one response expressed the dismay that they did not expect to come to a religious service!? Maybe this aspect of total health is

131

for more of us than we are prepared to admit, and the resistance to its implications of 'physician heal thyself' may lie in our inability to face our own humanness in our heroic desire to be the ones who 'fix it' for others.

24

PRACTICAL CARE IS SPIRITUAL CARE

At the basic level that most people experience the trauma of losing one's dignity in hospital is a much publicised issue. At present the media are concentrating on how elderly people and their relatives are quite upset about the levels of neglect that can sometimes occur in hospital wards and elderly care homes. Several years ago, having observed first- hand the state of some elderly patients' hair and nails, I wrote to the Head of Nursing pointing this out, and that just attending to these things might actually enhance the patient experience. Not surprisingly it did not happen, though I think the point I was making was understood. In the same way I suggested nurses should carry notebooks so they could note down patient requests rather than forgetting them due to overload. On another occasion, having been accosted in ICU by a very concerned family who had to pay a lot of money to park a long way away to see their seriously ill relative. In response I made an appointment to see the manager concerned. The issue had been identified. Something was done eventually to ease that family's burden. These are practical examples, but they can demonstrate that the hospital *cares*. After all most hospitals go to the trouble to have a flat or relatives room in the case of acute long stay patients, why not offer some designated parking close by. The support of relatives is so vital to their loved one's recovery.

Another area is that of feeding ill people who cannot easily do it for themselves. It is no wonder that there has been much in the press about neglect. Relatives are known to have become very upset when they discover un untouched place of food either within reach but uneaten, or slightly out of reach. Nurses do not always notice this, though they should, and often the efforts of relatives are not as welcomed as they should be. Protected Meal Times in hospitals may be all well and good, but they also act to keep away those who could help with the feeding of sick relatives.

One trainee nurse, it was reported, was asked to give a patient help with their food. Her response was "I've already done that" pointing to a tick in the box of her task sheet, as if a tick in the box designated the experience of feeding was what nursing was about. Nursing is about care. It is about people and their practical needs, and if five patients need help, then five people should receive that help. Enlisting families would go a long way to remedy this pressure.

GOOD PRACTICE

On the paediatric ward in my hospital the sight that first struck me is not just the row of sick or post operational young people but the array of gadgets like Nintendos and learning based computer programmes on offer as well as drawing and Lego type constructing aids. When you go on the ward the children and young people are often busy concentrating on stimulating school work and games. The thinking behind this is very practical but also sensitive to the situation. Imagine having a broken leg, or waiting for an operation with nothing to fill your time. The support teaching staff on these wards know that where there are energy levels there should be things to do. It also takes the sting out of waiting for the operation or the worries that can be around hospital stays with lots of tests and examinations, particularly if it takes time to make a diagnosis. It is also very helpful to parents who will otherwise have to spend a large amount of time with a bored child.

We used to have a Hospital School but it moved several years ago into the community. The idea was that young people should not lose out on their schooling when they had conditions or disabilities that required constant attention. These children were very much included in all the presentations that were done at the end of each term. It was a joy to see; so practical, but it constituted care of the tender human spirit of the disabled at the deepest level. It has to be said that many accidents and illnesses have a financial implication, if long term incapacity has to be faced. Care of any shape has to take these matters into consideration as a matter of course. Not to assess this area is a dereliction of duty, particularly as worries over money creates huge stress in a person's life.

One of my chaplaincy colleagues was really impressed whilst speaking to a middle-aged man with learning difficulties when someone else turned up from a day centre who was not a support worker or designated carer as such. This woman brought a bag with all kinds of things to do for this man, ranging from cross stitch to colouring in and drawing books. She also brought some sticker books. This woman was I believe, exercising a level of spiritual care in what she was doing. She may not have gathered that was what she was doing, but he did! The point is that it was so practical. Rather than coming along simply to talk or listen (when either activity might have been filled with some long silences) she released him from any anxiety that might have filled his time when he was sitting there doing nothing.

Some of the most effective ways of offering spiritual care - the therapy of that essential human within the patient - are the thoughtful and simple attentions we pay to their needs. It may be the provision of a newspaper to read to ease the boredom, or fetching some glasses without which the ward is a blur. It can be things like helping to write a card to a patient's friend, or saying a few prayers or even sitting with someone at the same time as a loved one's funeral is taking place. We have had a radio in our office donated to us that we have loaned out to patients who needed stimulation, but had no choice of what they could listen to. Although Roger Daltrey and countless other stars of the entertainment world may not realise it they contribute to the practical spiritual care of a particular category of cancer sufferer.

The Teenage Cancer Trust was set up to respond to the special requirements of children and young adults with cancer, who should rightly not be in paediatric or adult wards. They need something else in their experience of illness." Teenage cancer units aren't like ordinary cancer wards. Their home-from-home atmosphere helps create a sense of normality. The state-of- the- art units are bright and vibrant and will often include things like pool tables, jukeboxes, games consoles, computers and Webcams, ensuring they can keep in touch with family friends outside hospital. Alongside all this is a medical team of teenage cancer specialists whose knowledge creates a body of expertise that's second to none." (59)

A listener is someone who journeys alongside another. Sharing the suffering of another person on a journey of ill health is part of what holistic and spiritual care is all about. Over the years I have tried to pick up on people's practical needs. Many I have missed. There was the case of the glasses that transformed one patient's experience when she could finally *see* the ward and the nurses' faces. I also supplied a dying cancer patient with fruit juice, because it was only thing that brought her comfort and relief. The only reason I did this was that she mentioned it that often, that I could hardly not to it and sleep with a clear conscience afterwards!

THE EXTRA MILE THAT ALLEVIATES ANXIETY

A man with a serious back injury that disabled him had a tussle with the doctor over his return home to feed his birds. We spoke about this, and the situation was left that if he was not allowed home, I would do it for him. I probably should not have offered. There were boundary issues at stake here. However, a rare moment of the heart triumphing over the head that won the day. It might have been a better solution to contact the hospital social worker. However I did, and as things would have it, the doctor forbade him to leave the ward. He was clearly worried about his birds, having no family nearby to deal with them in his absence. He then armed me with diagrams of the aviaries, gave me the address and the combination to his alarm, which I had to deactivate to get at the keys to the aviaries. He had built these aviaries, so they were a bit like the Hampton Court Maze and rather difficult to negotiate.

I went to his home, and managed to get the keys and successfully get in the various aviaries. The different species of birds were kept in different parts of the construction which was in his front garden. I got the appropriate seed as described in his notes, fed them and also gave them water and carefully locked up afterwards. At the time I had a shaky feeling that I was probably taken on more than I should, and wished I had not been so hasty. Anyway, on my return, I assured him that his birds were just fine, and his relief was clearly visible. It was like a weight had been taken off his shoulders. I saw this action as a part of spiritual care. It is said that worries dispirit a person, therefore worry is a spiritual concern. His worry was addressed, though by doing it a few more were created for me!

WATER IN THE DESERT

It did not end there. I foolishly reminded him a week or so later that the water and food might have run out and so he insisted that I made a return visit. On that occasion I discovered to my horror that many of the birds were dead on the floor of the aviaries. I did not quite know how to break the bad news, but when he made enquiries after the welfare of his birds, I had to do the "well...er...um" routine and tell him. I thought he would be very angry, or suffer some reaction, but all he said rather casually was that when birds are moulting, they are prone to attack each other for some reason, as if it were common knowledge! Not all was lost then. At least I was able to get his benefit money from the Post Office with a letter of recommendation from him, and remind myself never to do this kind of thing again!

I first met Jessie when I was visiting her next bed neighbour Doris on the ward. Jessie indicated that she wanted to open up communication with me. Despite her desire to talk she did not come over as needy. She seemed a sweet, likeable lady. She soon shed tears as she related her story that was a recurrent theme of aloneness. "I am all alone in the world" were her own words.

She informed me that she was the last of a family of 10 children to survive. This meant she was used to many people around her all her life. This upbringing of constant noise and activity represented a huge contrast to her present ward experience. She had been married to two "grand men" - her words, but had survived them. Her only relative, by marriage, was Albert, her brother-in-law. He looked after her elderly dog, Princess. I can only describe her as generally cheerful, easy to be with, with simple wants and tastes, such as flowers around the ward and fruit drinks. With the recent decline in her health, apart from the pains that "really gripped her", she began to develop a craving for sharp tastes. At the same time she realised that the penalty for quenching her thirst was in fact that of being quite sick shortly after drinking. She was unselfconscious about this but is at the same time she was aware of the 'trouble' she thought it was causing nursing staff.

In our conversation she often broke down, especially when as she asked me to say a short prayer with her. The thing that brought her tears was that she felt forgotten especially when those who promised to do so did not fulfill their intentions by bringing her grapes that she so loved. She was upset when Albert forgot because in her words "he ought to remember". This upset her though she knew the grapes would probably not be kept down. Whilst there may have been other reasons for her sense of feeling alone such as being the last of the line with her nine siblings having died, I thought that along with the support she received from her adjacent bed neighbour Doris, she needed to feel heard and understood without having to ask. She knew she was very ill and that the end was not far away. She declined the offer of going to the nearby hospice. In that situation I did what I could including bringing her the fruit drinks she craved. She registered immense pleasure. Thereafter she received continuous pain control, but died quite suddenly. It may not seem much, but the practical supply of fruit drinks brought Jessie as much emotional and spiritual support as she was able to receive. The tangy flavours seemed to bring her a deep sense of comfort at her journey's end.

Journeys in life often contain strange meetings. Those synchronistic moments when we meet the right person at the right time, are a rare but welcome feature in the itinerary of life. Geoff was ending his travels, so to speak. He was a tall thin man in his late seventies giving all the impressions of strength and fitness. As I arrived in his area of the ward he exclaimed how extraordinary that I should turn up at this point. I took the cue and settled down into his bedside chair and prepared myself to listen.

He spoke of experiences earlier on in his life when he came down from the North-East with his family, as his father was seeking work. As a young lad with a beautiful singing voice he had won a scholarship to a choir school in the North-East when he was 12. He hoped to sing in the parish church when he moved south. He was welcomed with open arms. However when it came to long term commitment to the choir it was just not possible because his father's job then took them to live further out of town. Undaunted he turned up at the village church where eventually, after a few weeks singing in their choir the choirmaster announced "you can't sing" With that he was promptly dismissed from the choir which he had recently joined, shattering his confidence, being an outsider in the community. Being told he could not sing; that his voice was not up to it, was deeply confusing and hurt the young Geoff. It angered his family as well. It seemed that no one could right this wrong. So Geoff turned his back on the church until his years in the army. The grievance had struck deeply into his soul. He had harboured a lingering resentment about "a church that could allow such an injustice to go on under its nose". It was this that was troubling him when I walked onto the ward.

Coming to the end of his life he was facing the fact that nothing else could be done for him in terms of surgery. Being a person of some self- awareness, he wanted to put his affairs in order. This included this deep rejection that he considered that the church was responsible for. When he had shared this story as well as an 'out of body experience' which he felt no one else would really understand, he felt immense relief. Someone understood and didn't laugh at him. I accepted him his anger at his earlier rejection without attempting to minimise it. I also listened to his strange 'paranormal' experience without blinking. Actually, I heard many of these every year. I left him to move on in his last few weeks, hopefully with a burden shared and lightened. 'Being there', what we in our chaplaincy team record in our activity figures, is an important part of a ministry of presence, and a presence 'at the right time' for people is even more healing. In a way it is a very practical part of our role. Many health care professionals will see these things, but may not tie them in with a patient's deeper sense of well- being.

GIVING PERSPECTIVE

Whether it would be described as practical, I have discovered that there are many things that bring a sense of calm to patients. One such incident arose when I was visiting a man who had undergone gastric surgery. Terence had cancer and had recently undergone a painful operation. He was then experiencing post operational pain, and certainly could not have been described as thriving. Invasive operations do take a lot of time to get over. He had a drain and the resultant fluids were taking a long time to clear. Whilst he was generally fit he was also prone to being anxious. The problem is that Terence had been in hospital a long time, and that in itself, had closed him in upon his condition. He was in a dark place and all his body language conveyed this state of mind. Although he was nearly 60 he was keen to get back to an active lifestyle. He had somehow lost sight of the possibility of recovery simply because it had not happened in the time frame that he had expected.

After some visits I became very aware of his low state. Poor Terence still had various drips attached, and was struggling with quick movement. He really did seem depressed. For some reason I just felt that words were no longer what he needed. I had recently been on a short break to the Lake District and had bought a set of lovely photograph cards as a reminder of the area. I brought a card depicting a winding path up a hillside and offered it to Terence, and suggested he used it to visualise his future and 'get out' of the ward in his imagination. I thought no more about it, but actually the card had the effect of lifting his spirits. He loved the card. Even though the winding path of his recovery went into dips and valleys, I was able somehow to hold on to a hope for his eventual recovery, using the card as a visual reminder of that possibility.

Not long after I saw him at a summer fete for a hospital unit that was fundraising looking much fuller in the face and feeling much more hope about his future. Since then I have had small cards produced with rural or garden themes to offer patients when I felt it appropriate. Interestingly, pictures sometimes have the capacity to symbolise hope better than words. They seem to be able to spark something off within the individual that fuels the dormant spiritual fire of hope that lies within people when they are unwell. As with Terence the purpose is to get them beyond the four walls of their ward and the imprisonment that a long stay patient feels that they are experiencing. They had the function of giving perspective away from the limited hospital ward; a reminder of ill health.

25

THE HUMAN JOURNEY

I have often spoken of journeys. Pathways similarly are modern healthcare terms as used in 'Liverpool Care Pathway for the Dying Patient.' Developed over years through research and launched in 2009 this is a tool developed that enabled a process of identifying the patient who is nearing the end, and putting in place those things to make that time a more healing one. Although some concerns have been raised recently about the abuse of this plan, in regard to expediently hastening a person's natural end time, the original aim was for greater quality at this point in life. This picture of a journey is well used in Bedside Manna. It illustrates the onward movement of many aspects of life whether that of growing older, changing or the health pathway we all travel. The picture of human life as a journey can often be very helpful to people. The experience of ill health with its dips and troughs may be likened to a trek through the hills or journey through woods, fields and gullies in changing weather conditions, day and night. The bad times experienced when health fails are a part of the experience but not the whole of it. Every person has had a past that is important and a future, which may be uncertain, but nonetheless to be looked forward to. Coming into hospital often reduces all of this into an inescapable present from which there seems to be no way out. This all-pervading gloomy present is similar to holding a 5 pence coin at arm's length, where is seen in relation to the wider picture. Then if we hold it against our eye, it suddenly obliterates everything else as if it doesn't exist. Seen in context the coin is just one component of life; close against our eye it *is* our life. Our relationship with a person in accompanying them in this journey may help them see that this dark tunnel they are experiencing is only a stage in their life, and not the whole thing.

A recent past Chief Nurse Sarah Mulally is quoted in the Health Service Journal in an article by Jeremy Davies on spiritual and religious needs in patients that healthcare professionals and the organisation in which they work "need to recognise that in healthcare we join people on their life journey and for a time we travel with them." She comments further; "We need to better understand who they are and how we can work with them as partners on that journey. Central to this is understanding them as individuals who have many dimensions including a spiritual one." **(60)**

FINAL JOURNEYS

Another kind of journey was what one particular patient was planning. This was Megan who had leukemia. I spent a few hours with her in her single room before she went back onto the main ward and I continued to see her there. Megan was elderly and we talked about a lot of things. She was one of those people who it was easy to listen to. We spoke of family, health prospects and treatment among other things. The predominant topic of conversation was her wish to go back to Rothesay on the Isle of Bute just off the West Coast of Scotland where she was brought up. It was a pilgrimage that would take her back, not only to her roots but to see her old school friend and a cousin whom she was fond of.

Once we arrived at this topic of conversation, she was very willing to talk. She became more and more animated the more we discussed this project. Whilst Megan was quite winsome about this journey with all its promise, I wondered what function this had for her in a period when her health was clearly unequal to the hardship of such a long journey. I said nothing. On my penultimate visit, she began to talk quite openly about her death. This was a little surprising, as all the conversation about journeys and roots and old friends seemed to be avoiding this possibility. Not now. Although I was actually a relative stranger to Megan I marveled at how all of a sudden she was talking so freely. A barrier dropped.

On the last occasion I met with her, Megan was due to have further chemotherapy, but she was now allowing herself the possibility of *not* getting better. This time she got back to the subject of the trip to Bute, but she had realised this would not happen. I saw more clearly then that this journey supplied her with a dream to hold on to. Each section had been carefully mapped out, even the planning of what Travelodge she and her son would stay at. She now no longer needed that dream; it had served its purpose. Most significantly she told me she was feeling weak, that she had come to the end and did not want to 'try' any more. There would be no Rothesay - no Bute - no cousin and no journey. Responding to several cues, I gave her permission to feel the loss by just accepting what she said, and suggested that she might allow God to 'carry' her on the rest of the way. Up to that point there had been no particularly spiritual drift to our conversation, but it seemed very right then to both of us. She asked for a prayer. She died later that day, her journey over. She had let go.

'QUAILS'

Some journeys are very bumpy indeed. I believe there are people who have suffered greatly through ill health through no fault of their own. They need a mention. There are people whose life journeys just seem fraught with bad luck, hassles and deep sadness. They will just seem to the outsider to live life at the bottom of the pile. Many are regular visitors to hospitals. We developed the name 'quails' - not as any term of abuse but to reflect the pathos of their stories and their experiences. Many patients joke about being 'season ticket holders' because they are regularly showing up on the ward. This is especially true of those suffering from respiratory problems, where every turn in the weather and every cold seemed to compromise their breathing. These too fall within the quail category; though in fact they are precious human beings not birds!

Some time ago a colleague in the hospital went from a family occasion to a friend's house. After lunch this friend proudly took him to the splendid aviary at the bottom of the garden. There, he showed him some fabulous finches and canaries, all brightly coloured and very delicate. As my colleague gazed on the feathered delights flitting from branch to branch, he chanced to look down to the rather less glorious sight of some little quails darting to and fro on the ground. He mused to himself that these little flightless birds had a poor lot in life, as they were in the line of fire from above and treading through the finch droppings below. There was no escape. From this encounter the term 'quails' originated for us. It came to describe those who often came into hospital, seemingly put upon from every angle in life, often victims of sheer bad luck. We met with them often. Each had their tale to tell, and few were self- pitying or especially angry with life. Bad things happen to all people, even 'good people'. Can we make any sense of it? They certainly couldn't? We were impressed at the way some people do cope in great adversity. In some ways these 'quails' had a lot going for them.

Eddie was a 'quail'. He had all sorts of medical complications and made many approaches to the Health Service, experiencing a whole range of responses and treatment. Being a doctor himself did not really seem to help him in all this, as he sought support, diagnosis, treatment and understanding. He described to me how he felt like a pariah within the profession precisely because he had been a medical practitioner and was ill long term. It was almost as if he were letting the side down. Despite numerous visits to several different hospitals over a number of years, no one seemed to be able to help him. There was little empathy around with what he had gone through. All manner of things were wrong with him and he was fortunate that his partner Catherine was very devoted in supporting him.

Chronic pain was the worst of his symptoms. This pain appeared not to respond to any interventions. Maybe the hardest thing for any doctor to face is being the chronic sufferer who just does not seem to get any better. He was an intelligent and interesting man, who had a lot to give. He was bedbound now and the prognosis was bleak. The medical professional does not always sit comfortably with anything that smacks of failure. Perhaps the specialists who could not cure him felt that failure. Care should be there even when there in no cure. I had to ask myself the question when does a reluctance to take personal responsibility for a long term patient, who may not get better, border on neglect. Sadly Eddie died. I am sure he felt let down by all who attended him. As a 'quail' he was not bitter, but he did feel some of the specialists insinuated that somehow his condition was his fault. I think the long term sick sometimes do feel this. We only have to look at the way ME, the post viral syndrome, has had to fight its corner to be acknowledged as a legitimate medical condition, in much the same way as shell shock used to be seen as cowardice in World War 1 and is now recognised as Post Traumatic Stress Disorder. The term 'malingerer' tended to follow sufferers of this condition in the early days.

'Quails' (who are actually real people who feel deeply, with family members anxious about them) are one of the greatest challenges to our ability in the NHS to care. Those who simply don't get better can be a frustration to our grandiosity. We have a need to learn that there are some things in life we simply cannot control.

26

THE STRENGTH IN HELPLESSNESS

The 'quail' factor increases our sense of being helpless in being close to the plight of the frequently ill. Incredulity is one common accompaniment to witnessing such suffering that seems to have no end; we can't believe it. Another is the way it points to what we cannot solve. We are helpless in the face of realities bigger than ourselves. Maybe the doctors who attended Eddie felt helpless in the light of his intractable medical condition. Those who generally have success in treating people may find that when the situation that will not resolve it is an offence to their profession. We are not in healthcare to exert power over patients, but to serve them with compassion, expertise and understanding. Sometimes that will require humility in the face of suffering. However helplessness is not the same as uselessness. We think it is which is why we try to avoid it. As we shall see to share in a feeling of helplessness with another may be very healing in itself.

During a Major Incident, many gallons of hot tea will be made for relatives by staff and volunteers. Behind this obvious act of kindness and consideration lies the fact that when faced with the pain of the unspeakable we find our own helplessness just too much. To do *something*, be it making a cup of tea makes us feel more useful. The same actions may well be replicated up and down the country in Police Stations, Funeral Director's reception areas and Mortuaries. The sight of a couple with pale and numbed expressions with their hands clasped round a steaming mug is an all familiar sight in these places of trauma. However, this comment is not intended to be a slight on the tea makers; I have done it myself as relatives have come into the reception areas after such a disaster. The fact of the matter is that we *are* often helpless in the face of some events. This action works both ways. We feel better, and the tea is a kindness offered which is also therapeutic. To give another something comforting and warm to hold when their senses have temporarily closed down is probably the best help we can give at that time.

We shouldn't think that it is patients or relatives that have the monopoly on these helplessness feelings. Everyone does; from the department who experience three stillbirths in a week and call in emotional support, to those manning the phone lines during the Alder Hey Tissue Retention scandal of 2001. Where do the professionals put their reaction to others' anger, grief and sense of betrayal? A feeling of powerless in hospital affects many people. For a patient it can feel that everything is happening *around* us, and we are somehow not part of it. These are all more common experiences than we would wish. Imagine the helplessness that many parents themselves experience at a late miscarriage, stillbirth or having a premature baby being treated in the Special Care Baby Unit. All they can do is to be deeply anxious, sick to the stomach, numb and even angry. If it is part of their usual pattern of response to the unimagineable, some will say a silent prayer and just hope against hope. Something that is 'out of our hands' is always so difficult to face. Chaplains, volunteer visitors and relatives, as well as nursing and medical staff will also feel impotent at times. A hospital is the kind of environment when being in control can seem unattainable from time to time. Feeling these things is an unnerving experience, but it does not always have to be the last word in failure. In feeling helpless ourselves, we can sometimes be in a better position to come alongside a patient than coming with platitudes and false hope.

Many a chaplain or volunteer visitor will come away from a patient contact feeling that they had nothing to say or no word of comfort or consolation. It may have been deep tears of brokenness and despair that prompted this, or may be the result of hearing bad news. The result is that the listener feels that they have nothing to say which may not sound glib, patronising or just empty. The result is a kind of dominant feeling of helplessness. Far from being failure, this staying with the patient under these circumstances and sharing that experience of powerlessness with them, is in fact a strength to them; often more than we realise.

THE STORY THAT LEAVES YOU SPEECHLESS

As with the history of the 'quails', so there are people we meet whose stories leave us speechless. Heinrich greeted me as I met him one day with an impromptu commentary on the state of the world. He seemed troubled and embittered, and reacted to me at the beginning. As I eventually came to see, the sight of my clerical collar had triggered a whole shower of negative emotions in him. Heinrich was certainly angry and bewildered that the world had not turned out the shape he wanted it to be. All the changes that had happened to him in an alien culture as well as experiencing ill health seemed just too much. A German, now resident in England and in his seventies, he gave vent to a flow of feelings and I just had to sit down and listen. As is turned out, I really had no answers. I sensed that was not what he was after anyway, just a willing ear.

After an hour or so he certainly seemed to have gained a greater peace within himself. He then thanked me for listening. Later on in the corridor I met his named nurse and she remarked that Heinrich had not stayed so still since he had been admitted. He was so jumpy and restless. The next day I happened to meet him elsewhere in the hospital, and he greeted me with a sense of knowing recognition and we exchanged nods.

Heinrich had a harrowing story of wartime adventures and troubles. It began with his entry into the Hitler Youth movement with great idealism which ended up after a prank that went wrong in being drafted the Russian Army. It was a mind boggling story, like a film. There then followed torture and a mock execution when a gun was placed to his head while blindfolded. This callous treatment was followed by a term in a Siberian labour camp. He met some wonderful people in the hell of that existence, had some kind of spiritual awakening there. Unlike many of his friends he did manage to return home.

The crux of his trouble with me was that in Germany at that time there was a Church tax; everyone pays. One of the first communications he had with the outside world on his return to his home town was a tax demand in person from the Church for the time he had been away! Just imagine his feelings. No wonder my clerical collar evoked his initial reaction. This is a poignant example of the fact that most people in hospital have their stories. Maybe not all stories are as shocking and eventful as extraordinary as Heinrich's. As Henri Nouwen has observed, "But when we take the word diagnosis in its most original and profound meaning of knowing through and through (*gnosis*/knowledge; *dia*/through and through), we can see that the first and most important aspect of all healing is an interested effort to know patients fully, in all their joys and pains, pleasures and sorrows, ups and downs, highs and lows, which have given shape and form to their life and have led them through the years to their present situation." (61)

The NHS of course does not exist primarily to hear our stories but for patients they do offer a clue to their lives and sometimes their health. As Dietrich Bonhoeffer, a German pastor and theologian who was executed the day after the war ended observed, it is not just a matter of what a person has done or not done in their life that should carry our judgment, but understanding for what they have suffered. Heinrich had certainly suffered deep trauma. That was a key to who he had become. I cannot say I felt anything other than helpless listening his story and the strength of his feelings. I shared some small responsibility for the unfeeling nature of the German Church at that time. Thankfully I managed to stay with it; which was all that was required for Heinrich to get something major off his chest.

The many Volunteer Chaplaincy Visitors we train up to add support on the wards invariably report back at our in-service training sessions that they feel very helpless when people share their pain. This is almost a necessary step for all of us walking 'where angels fear to tread'. We often have to tell them that it is all right to feel helpless as the patient will almost certainly feel that themselves. There is nothing worse than feeling absolutely awful, vulnerable, isolated and anxious *and* on top of it all then have some hearty individual jollying you along. More than likely, false heartiness will make you feel very much worse or even like hitting them! When someone visits you in vulnerability, you may be more likely to feel a sense of accompaniment. Someone who can pick up your cues, with no easy answers to give is a welcome solace, bedside manna even!

A sensitive hospital visitor like anyone in the acute health setting, may be the better for having their own areas of vulnerability. We all have our wounds, open or healing, but all that makes us is human.

Annie Sullivan who was known for her remarkable work with the deaf and blind girl Helen Keller, celebrated in the film 'The Miracle Worker', had her own handicaps. Far from disabling her from being an agent of change and support, it helped her all the more to enter into the isolated world of this lonely girl, cut off from others and angry with the world. So it is with all of us, these wounds and scars we pick up in life may actually count among our gifts; our passport into the lives of others, whom the 'fit and able' cannot reach!

BREAKING BAD NEWS

There is another side to communications that need regular attention in hospital. The breaking of bad news is probably something most doctors would wish not to have to do. Many have to. Over the years I have seen the brilliant and sensitive handling that some clinicians bring into this difficult area. You can often see as patients and relatives will tell you, that when they were informed of what they had been dreading, it was done with great care and a truly empathetic manner. The feeling of powerlessness is present on both sides in that situation. Feeling the patient and family's numbness and helplessness and acknowledging it in ourselves, usually makes us better bearers of bad news.

I marvelled on one occasion as an oncologist was communicating on a sensitive area with someone I knew quite well from my last parish experience. I was with her when the doctor arrived with some test results. I never got the chance to show my appreciation to him for how he treated her; though I made a point of trying to coincide with him on the ward. Perhaps he might have found it patronising. The opposite happens too, and patients have voiced their disgust to me at hearing examples of the insensitive handling of delicate moments. The curtains round the beds don't always muffle the goings on inside them. Particularly negligent I feel is the habit leaving a patient alone after delivering a verbal knock-out blow. I have been the next to visit after this event on several occasions, and have had to pick up the pieces.

However I heard from someone recently that their father was awaiting the results of some tests, and the doctor walked to his bedside and said, "You only have weeks to live." The whole family was totally devastated. Firstly they were not expecting it, and secondly the brusque and unfeeling manner in which this startling news was conveyed was not appropriate to the situation. When the doctor left the room one of the family rushed out and expressed strongly how badly the doctor had handled this. In response the doctor, a young man in his thirties, turned round and said, "I am only doing my job." If that were true, then it seems to me that he was either the wrong person for the job, or had not been trained well enough to deal with this most crucial of encounters. He was not certainly dealing with the helplessness he may well have been feeling himself underneath it all, or that of the patient. Who does train people for this skill? Perhaps only life does. Is the feeling of impotence in the course of delivering medical expertise addressed in Medical or Nursing School? Embracing a level of helplessness in the face of difficulties should be addressed without disempowering healthcare staff as this skill can actually be a strength for people, not a weakness. Of course it needs to be recognised, that in hospital for the most part, there is the breaking of good news too!

As a rider to this section, I believe there should be routine attention within the field of pre-assessment for operations and also cancer and other life threatening conditions concerning what *might* happen. Pre-assessments are often thorough, but perhaps in some respects not thorough enough. In the roller coaster of hearing a difficult diagnosis, particularly if it is out of the blue, or indeed a 'worst case scenario' people need emotional preparation alongside the usually efficient and thorough physical preparation. Patients may need to hear whether they are likely to come off better or worse after a particular intervention. They may need to put on to specific support groups for their condition. Surely hospital staff would want all of these things for themselves should that moment come. It may be an area where angels fear to tread but it is necessary; and I suspect from the horror stories I have been told, a very patchy aspect of patient preparation. People are not ready for blunt pronouncements, they are tender plants and require treating as such.

Who shares in this helplessness around?

When the question is asked, "who should do this work?" The simple answer is that everyone can to one degree or another. Rabbi Julia Neuburger hits the nail on the head. She writes; "But in fact spiritual care goes much wider than chaplaincy. It is not only chaplains who provide it. It can, and often is, provided by every member of the healthcare team, if they have the sensitivity and skills, as well as other staff members, particularly the cleaning and portering staff, who often, by their very common sense and willingness to talk where health staff fear to tread, provide some of the best spiritual care settings in this country." (62) We may also ask; "What are the qualifications for doing this well?" Again, the answer is that far from academic and professional qualifications being the key, experience of life, particularly through those events that have hurt and caused vulnerability constitute some of the raw materials that help to develop warm empathy and compassionate engagement with others.

Alistair V. Campbell (not Tony Blair's one time Press Secretary) wrote a book "Paid to Care?" (63) In his book Campbell sets out to explore the limits of professionalism in pastoral care. He also begs the obvious debate about the vocational aspect of nursing. A person who cares will inevitably do so because of who they are. You don't become caring all of a sudden just by being paid to support sick or vulnerable people. It is the other way round; you do a caring job because you care. It is part of you. Though we have to be aware of the temptation in caring to try and 'rescue' people or situations. We tend to do this mostly because we can't stand the feeling of helplessness in ourselves and want to solve things for our sake as much as the other person. What happens when that other person isn't or cannot be rescued? Beware!

The lie is lent to the notion that all healthcare workers are going to be willing to share in the understanding treatment of the vulnerable. I was told of a worrying incident a few weeks ago, where a 92 year old woman, partially sighted but sound of other faculties, was attending an eye clinic in a London hospital. Having been taken there by the taxi company she knew, and treated with exemplary courtesy and skill by the medical staff for her condition, she needed to return home. She informed the reception where she was sitting after her treatment if they could get her familiar taxi for her. She had her usual firm in her mind, but was abruptly told by the receptionist that she knew the numbers required and would this woman take her seat. Whether the receptionist had picked up on her partially sighted difficulty and the effect this had or not, nothing happened. So half an hour later this woman asked the receptionist how things were going with the taxi only to be told briskly that it was not a taxi but a porter that was being summoned. A name like hers was called out as next in line and when she queried the name, she was informed it was not her. A moment or two later the name was repeated but the full name was then given. When the porter did arrive, this woman was taken outside, shown a telephone and told to order a taxi. When the woman told him that she could not see to make the call, there was a reluctant pause, a call was made and she was told that she was number 18 in the queue. All the while this treatment seemed to reinforce the feeling for this vulnerable lady that she was a nuisance, and saddest of all, that she was not valued or supported as someone in need. This, surely is not a health inducing response, and does much to increase the feeling of helplessness and anger in the patient. It also makes me query the training staff receive.

CARING FOR THE CARERS

Even if we are caring and compassionate people the pressures can become too great if we don't keep our boundaries of self-care. It is no failure to know our own limits. Burnout with its attendant 'withdrawal' from others' human need occurs regularly in healthcare. The greatest cause of sickness and absence in healthcare employees is actually put down as stress, although the figures won't define what kind of stress is involved. Doctors and nurses are subject to all the vulnerabilities that their patients are, and it is a gross misconception that the 'helping personality' is somehow above these facts of life.

The question for today is whether the standards of care have actually dropped because nursing may be seen by some people as just a job, irrespective of the emotional and physical cost that caring demands of the individual. Personally I believe it makes sense that if a person is drawn toward any form of caring/helping profession because it probably ties in with their general draw towards helping others. It is similar to a person who is good with their hands and has a firm grasp of physics or mechanics who might be drawn to training to be an electrician or a plumber. I need to make the point that simply being paid is unlikely to automatically trigger something that is not programmed into that person from the outset. We still need training before and during our work to keep our skills and insight on the up and not becoming in danger of stagnating! All innate gifts and abilities need further honing. There are really no examples in life of the 'finished product'!

This perception is illustrated by a recent shocking Panorama report in June 2011 about the physical and emotional abuse that took place in private care homes for people with learning disabilities. I wonder whether a frustration for some people develops precisely because of the feelings of helplessness felt when patients cannot or do not engage with their treatment. The temptation to control or even bully can go hand in hand with frustration. Patients are after all only people just like us; we have to try to understand them, using our own understanding of ourselves as a way of getting into the experience of others. It is what empathy is all about. There is no reason why empathy should not contain feelings of helplessness. If that feeling of helplessness is present in the other person, then it could be a help in supporting them.

A vocational approach to health care professions may seem rather idealistic in today's world, but if looking after others is not a heart thing as well as a professional and practical thing, I am led to wonder how far people will be prepared to go in the care and comfort of others. When the presently intense pressures in the wards, clinics and theatres get to find the chinks in people's emotional and physical armoury, then breakdown may possibly follow. Work related stress as well as outside pressures can contribute to much of the sick leave in hospital staff these days. I think a health warning needs to be given to many public services these days, not just for nursing and doctoring, but the police, fire, and social services.

Several years ago I attended a helpful day conference put on by the Accident and Emergency Department of a large city hospital. The title was 'The Emotional Cost of Caring'. The assumption in the title was that looking after others in tense situations in the long term, took its toll. We came from different wings of the caring professions, but we all saw that we had many things in common. At times it felt like an unrelenting task to care for others, but we had to be willing to pay the price. We also discovered we needed to attend to our own needs. Heroism was not called for in helping professions, common sense was. Among the feelings many of us experienced as we shared that day was the one of feeling powerless at times. On reflection but this was probably nothing in comparison to what those we cared for were feeling.

27

THE FINAL CURTAIN

No treatment of holistic, pastoral, and spiritual care in a health care setting would be appropriate without the recognition of our mortality. Although aspects have been looked at in Chapter 24 there are further pastoral and spiritual angles on this mystery of life. From middle age onwards we may find we are aware that things are not how they used to be, and the capacity to bounce back from illness has diminished through the years. The pathway of dying is something that different people face in different ways. We need to allow people to explore this within their own limits. Accepting other people's tolerances around the subject of death is kind and caring, and enables them to proceed on this journey with all the support that they may need. Life is incredibly precious, more so when it is threatened. No wonder most of us hang on to it at all costs.

Many people over the years have been very direct to me about dying. Equally, I have sensed the downward spiral that may occur just before death, when the patient is making resolute noises about getting better. People vary. However, the ones who speak in a direct manner often want a response. Sometimes they want to shock, because their prognosis is a shock to them. It is like they want to know what effect such devastating news will have on a third party, particularly a chaplain who may be expected to say words of profound meaning to uplift the 'condemned' person. Many others I have found are in hospital shortly after the death of a loved one. This recent bereavement may be a hidden stress that somehow weakens the immune system. It is uncanny just how often a reference is made to a close member of the family, particularly a partner or spouse, who has left a gaping hole in the life of that person. When a death is felt consciously or otherwise by a patient as an 'amputation', a period of emotional draining and instability often arises during which that person is somehow disconnected. This, in my experience of listening, I feel is prime territory for heart problems

156

and falls, particularly when people are elderly. As people who try to care, with an eye for the whole person, this area of recent loss should capture our special attention.

Personally, I am very grateful that a person wants to speak out when what is happening to them must be deeply painful. I want to help them to live with the recognition that something final may soon have to be faced, and yet there is still much to do in living out those final months, weeks, and days. Working on a haematology ward where patients undergo chemotherapy, I noticed how each individual reacts differently. The clinicians have to arrange slightly different medication for each new person, and monitor how they do with it. There is a difference in the pattern of diseases such as leukemia from one person to another. Some get through it and return to get back to normal living again. Others do well and then later on have a second spell when remission gives way to illness and they go downhill quite rapidly.

Walking the ward may feel sometimes like negotiating the route of eggshells. In fact the opposite is often true. There can be quite an atmosphere of reality amid the very mixed fortunes of leukemia sufferers. It is worse when bad news comes out of the blue. On one occasion I happened upon a patient whom I had been seeing for the best part of a year, on and off. I entered his room to find the family in great distress as they had been told them he only had weeks left, when he appeared to have made some remarkable progress. I have to admit I was as stunned as they were, and had to sit down. I found myself weeping. There was nothing helpful that I could say. As I was the only one in tears I felt that I have been became a channel for the family's grief as they were too stunned to own their deepest feelings at that point. In fact being the next person to visit a patient who has just learned some unwelcome news has become strangely common in hospital visiting on the wards.

I have referred already to the fact that a patient should not be left alone after bad news unless they have requested it. Feelings of numbness, shock and disbelief often come before those of sadness or anger. When and if acceptance comes that can be a healing moment. Such is the pressured environment of the NHS ward of today that it is not always possible to for a doctor to stay around and provide this pastoral consideration. Being an independent person arriving between the patient's comprehension of what feels like a death sentence and their inevitable choice whether to tell the family immediately, can lead them to a degree to acceptance. If they want to they can bounce their thoughts off someone who isn't medical, and isn't family. Many have done that with me. Often the truth does not sink in until a person's nearest relatives can share that difficult reality together. People vary in their reaction to bad news as widely as they vary in their attitude to their possible death. I am not sure the NHS or its staff deals particularly well with this. It does take time and patience, two things that can be in short supply in busy wards. Death may also feel like a negation of all they do. Hospitals are there to preserve life, after all. They are places for healing, surely. We need to remember that a huge number of people do die in hospitals. People will often discern when the time has come for a loved family pet to be put out of its suffering and whilst feeling bad about doing it, have them put down. We can't do that very easily to human beings, but we can help people die with dignity.

For some time on one particular ward elderly people would tell me that they wanted to die. For the most part that was an accurate summary of how it felt for them. They were tired, they had had enough. An uncomfortable and invasive procedure was about to be done to them and they simply did not want it. On some occasion neglect was a part of this expression of feeling. One day I was paged whilst in the hospital and was asked by the ward staff to visit an elderly lady who wanted to see "a priest". Having checked that it was not a Roman Catholic priest they needed I proceeded up to the ward. Her name rang a bell with me, and when I saw her I was familiar with her as a frequent visitor. This is not uncommon for a Respiratory ward, where many repeat visits when breathing becomes impossible or they get a chest infection. She proceeded to inform me that she wanted to die. She was due a procedure for which she required a partial anaesthetic, but she was very uncertain that it would improve her quality of life. I felt she was brave to tell me, but I informed her that I did hear what she was saying and recognised her tiredness and readiness to die. Her affairs were in order and she had no children. I said I could not help her to do this legally, nor could the hospital, but with her permission I would say a little prayer with her and visit her the next day. The nurse greeting me outside the ward was clearly concerned with the turn this lady's condition was taking, and I think expected me to "talk her out of it". That is never a part of our support. If people know their own minds, they need to be given the dignity of being understood and affirmed; although in the case of a strong desire to die, not too robustly!

A man in terrible suffering because of a lung complaint also said something similar to me. It was veiled, but I caught his meaning. I said to him, "I wish for you what you would wish for yourself". One day after a Sunday Chapel Service elsewhere in the Trust I was contacted by pager to attend to this man. The family was also present there. I felt that I was able to echo his deepest desires in my prayer at the bedside, and took his funeral service a week later. Why should we want to control how adults feel when they clearly possess little quality of life? Many are actually are ready to move on into the uncertainty of death. Compared with how they are feeling, it would seem a reasonable gamble for them. I think it takes courage to face these issues, and in some ways they are easier to address when hearing an open admission of wanting to die with than when a person who is critically ill and is in denial about it.

LAST RIGHTS?

Apart from the right of a very poorly person to make a Living Will and post a Do Not Resuscitate clause in their patient notes, patients can and do have some control over their last moments.

There are also questions asked in health care today about the best place to die. People are very different about this. Even the manner of a person's death can vary according to the personality concerned. I visited one lady at the request of her daughters as I knew them from dealing with the family over the final days and the death of their father. When this lady eventually died, it was not when they were present, which they would have preferred, but exactly when they had gone for a tea break. It seemed that she chose not to inflict this event on them. They eventually saw that it was 'just like their mum' to do that. Another elderly lady had been in the Burns Unit for some time. When I visited one afternoon her friend was there. We sat together saying little while the disturbed breathing of the dying lady was telling us that she had little time left. At a certain point a nurse came in with some flowers for her. She was unconscious. The flowers came with a note that her nephew who lived abroad, was thinking of her, as she was unmarried, this nephew represented her next of kin, her closest tie. Within moments of our reading the card to her she died. I like to think that she was hanging on for this recognition from her nephew. It was uncanny. Her friend and I looked at each other, wondering if she had 'hung on' for this news.

A SAFE PLACE

Different personalities and temperaments in people may well dictate where they may feel their last moments should come. Oncology departments, along with MacMillan nurses try to gather whether a person would be happiest to die at home. What does that person want? How does the family feel about it? Is there sufficient support? Is it safe? We are all familiar with films and paintings where a touching bedside scene depicts a dying matriarch or patriarch with all their family present. At one time this may have been the only option. Circumstances and our culture have changed since those times. There are other options today. Sadly, I believe we are all ready to consign extremely ill people to strangers in unfamiliar surroundings at a point of extreme frailty. It is possible that the move in itself might hasten death. Would we want to be driven in an ambulance and undergo all the stress and uncertainty involved when we are barely clinging on to life? I am sure most families try and do their best for their relatives, but I wonder whether our own reluctance to face the last journey ourselves is a factor in getting them off our hands and let the professionals deal with them?

That is a cynical view perhaps, but we do not on the whole embrace death as part of life. Cristina Odone comments; "Our culture treats death as a taboo. As a result, few, even among health professionals, can diagnose when someone is dying, relieve their pain, and help reconcile them to their inevitable fate. Care home staff, GPs unfamiliar with the patient's history, family: again and again, their first instinct is to rush the patient to hospital. Fifty eight per cent of Britons die in an NHS ward." (64) We need to think about this and perhaps be willing to ask the seriously ill person what they would like. Allowing ourselves to be exposed to a higher level of emotional pain than we want, might be the price we pay for letting someone end their days among those who love them. This though may be the best spiritual care we can give.

A new awareness around the process of death has entered the field of the support of the dying in the form of 'soul midwives' where death is recognised as a much a necessity of life as birth. That being the case, the soul midwife helps the person who requires their presence and support to make that final journey with a companion similar to some mothers-to-be who may require the services of a 'doula' who supports them in a non-medical way. These people in no way want to take people from their family setting, any more than the doula may want to *compete* with midwives. It is about emotional and spiritual support at a very important, and often fearful time of life. For those who are aware enough at the approach of death, it can be very helpful to be told "You are doing so well," in the same way as a mother-to-be needs encouragement during the birth of a baby "A good death is an extraordinary, moving and sacred experience. It can also have a healing quality, not only for the person who is involved but their families, friends and the wider community" is the view of Felicity Warner who pioneers this form of support. (65)

The tendency for some people who are nearing the end time, is to get things off their chest. It may be an extreme example and an extraordinary time to do this, but more than one person has divulged that they had been sexually abused in their early life when nearing their final hours. There was little doubt that this disclosure, painful as it was, helped them to move on in the knowledge that it was a difficult experienced believed by a third party, and was now 'out in the open'. One gentleman called me out at night to confess how badly he had treated his family during his lifetime. The only problem was that he had failed to tell his assembled family that this was the reason that a chaplain was visiting him late at night when he had no previous involvement with the Church. The confession happened in an informal way and I heard it informally, and reflected that I was maybe not the person to be telling. I ran the gauntlet of the bemused members of his family on the way out, and couldn't really tell them anything.

As we have to point out on our Grief and Loss training in the hospital, the death of a loved one is not the only source of loss in life. All kinds of situations create a sense of loss, and we have to learn to be aware what we are feeling and give ourselves time to work through it. Others may have to stay with us on this uncomfortable journey, and that takes great sensitivity. To give examples, apart from someone's death, or a pet's death to children and adults, the severity of the feelings of loss may relate to the manner of that death and the relationship of that person to you, and any history that goes with along with it. There are also the losses of relationship breakdown, moving house or job, children leaving home, growing old, and the loss of a feeling of safety when your house is burgled. Those who have suffered spinal or brain injuries or who have had strokes will "lose" the life they once had, with all the symptoms of bereavement that go with it.

The death of a parent or a partner, or someone particularly significant if you have learning disabilities like a support worker, will have wider ramifications than we might imagine. There we have the situation of multiple losses. In these situations a move from your home may be involved along with the absence of a meaningful other. Accompanying these, there may be the loss of familiar surroundings, a secure routine of life and a network of relationships. This may not be clear whilst the personal grief is strongly present, but these things may figure in the support people need after a death, from those closest to them or involved with them professionally.

However cancer patients particularly will recognise another set of significant losses in their journey through diagnosis and treatment. Sometimes we forget how much a person's world changes when undergoing the undignified side effects of chemotherapy for instance. The patient in serious illness may well have to face some of the following losses:

loss or threat to self-image

loss of bodily integrity

loss or interruption to work

loss of independence

loss of dignity

loss of identity

loss or threat to cognitive functioning

loss/threat to a future

loss/strain on relationships

loss of sexual expression

loss of faith

This is a hefty list, and the same resources needed to face the death of a person you loved may have to come into play when people face these issues, even temporarily. It takes some empathy to know and see what people are going through, so as not to minimise their experience or treat them as somehow 'feeble' when they express emotion about them. Life is all about losses. This is how we all have to grow and develop. The baby loses something to become a toddler, who loses to face the challenges of school and so on. This will never change, we just have to be aware of our own losses and be willing to face them in order to be realistic about those of others.

28

WHAT NEXT . . .?

Ill health is bad enough. Accidents cannot always be avoided. Both require thorough medical attention, and often further support from the therapies in aftercare. However, trauma is seldom far away from the patient experience, but I believe and have tried to demonstrate from the priorities of changing times and from many examples of the patient experience that this widespread trauma is not factored in as I believe it should be. An example of this was when I once offered my services to all the critical and trauma care departments a few years ago, having done some critical incident debriefing training. Having spent NHS money on training I wanted to make it count. They were all more than happy to give time to listen to me. They saw the possibilities and the support it could bring. When it came to it, by the lack of further response none of them saw a place for my regular work with patients. Did they forget? Was it not a priority? Were the few clinical psychologists that there were the only ones there professionally able to help? Was something missing in their awareness of the patients need, I wonder?

Frank Parkinson in his book 'Coping with Post-Trauma Stress', defines post trauma stress as "The development of characteristic symptoms following a psychologically distressing event outside the range of normal human experience." **(66)** As he lists some of the 'major incidents' that may contribute to this, amongst the more high profile ones such as natural or man-made disasters, shootings, bombings and terrorist activity and fatal accidents, he draws attention to some less extreme examples. But these are traumatic in their way although their effects may go unnoticed because they are not so obvious or dramatic. Under this heading we find physical and emotional abuse, bullying of any kind, miscarriages, abortions and stillbirths, bereavement, marital distress, being given bad news of a death, serious disease or terminal illness. The hypothesis in this book clearly adds the additional trauma of illness and a stay in hospital. These examples that Parkinson highlights are not far away from the stories people will tell us in hospital. Trauma not only needs to be acknowledged but responded to appropriately.

At the risk of repeating myself, I question whether the NHS has really grasped the nettle regarding the complementary need for the pastoral side of medicine in the hospital setting. Doctors, nurses and health professionals vary enormously in their perception of what constitutes good care. Many exercise excellent pastoral and spiritual care in their concern and manner of handling different patients and their needs. But I have also heard lip service paid to the subject at the highest levels, but it has not formally translated into action. Is it simply too costly? Does it not tick any of the Care Quality Commission's boxes? Whilst I may think that spiritual care of the whole person is quality care because I am a chaplain, many others may argue that people come to hospital to get 'fixed', and when this is done the hospital has achieved its purpose.

Chaplaincies vary too. Some may have full support of the Trust and be given resources to be a viable presence, added that bit extra to a person's experience of the system. Other Chaplaincy services exist as trace elements only, responding only to crisis intervention, and run any religious requirements patients and staff may have. In those situations chaplains are run off their feet because on-call requirements with one or two chaplains leave little time for recovery. In our most chaplain rich era, we had a staff of 19, whole-time and part-time along with a paid part-time secretary. We also held the Line Management of Bereavement Services as the Department of Health specified as appropriate. It is a vastly different situation that prevails today six years later. After at least rounds of budget cuts, and as well as the move of Bereavement Services to other management structures we now have half the staff that we had in 2005, and the likelihood is that the Service will no longer be led by a Head of Department, but be transferred to another Line Manager who is not a chaplain. In fairness all Departments have taken a hit with the various rounds of cuts, ours is not singled out, though it does represent a disinvestment in spiritual care. I am only too aware of budgetary restraints in the NHS, but I wonder what signals this sends out to the community who are in the know about these things and whether in time the pendulum may swing back the other way, as nursing staff are looked to more and more for the pastoral and spiritual support many need in hospital.

CARING FOR THE SPIRIT

When the College of Healthcare Chaplains and the Department of Health had a concerted attempt to strengthen the pastoral, religious and spiritual side of medicine in the early 2000s, there were raised hopes that the issues of a deeper patient care was being recognised by the NHS. Several publications in 2003, such as 'Caring for the Spirit' (CHCC 2003) and 'Chaplaincy: meeting the Religious and Spiritual needs of Patients and Staff' (Department of Health 2003) highlighted the importance of spiritual care. In addition CHCC outlined a new job structure as well as selection and training procedures for chaplains. However there was little money to support these bold initiatives so that nearly ten years later the Service round the country is as patchy as ever. Many resultant initiatives such as local Spiritual Healthcare Collaboratives came and went, as pressures within the Health Services prohibited time out and ready access to travelling expenses. It was not all bad news. One such Collaborative seems to have succeeded in getting spiritual care more robustly back into the University syllabus for nurse training. The whole area of Research in spiritual care also found its way onto the agenda in these years. Over the Border the Scottish NHS on the other hand did in fact provide funding and the matter of chaplaincy and pastoral, religious and spiritual support has been systematically addressed in a more positive way. I am personally grateful for their pioneering work. In fact the NHS over the border enabled our own service to draft a Holistic and Spiritual Healthcare Policy in 2004, using the templates that each NHS area authority provided. Ultimately the Trust adopted a Policy that looked similar to what was already in place in Scotland.

In some ways part of the problem with a more comprehensive approach to patient care, is discerning what lies beneath the more obvious health issues. Underneath is the need for a more full blooded acknowledgement that patients are people and that ill health and hospitalisation create anxiety. At various levels as we have seen, it is traumatic. People worry about their health. Common questions might be what a diagnosis might be, what procedures will be used, "will it hurt; will I get better?" We have established that worry dispirits people, so worry is a spiritual need. Because hospitals are breeding grounds for anxiety, this constitutes a legitimate need for spiritual care alongside clinical intervention. Today our health system is creaking at the seams. Nursing staff have more and more asked of them, and at more responsible levels than thirty years ago. Nurse training expects less ward time of students than before with the result that the experience of working with ill and sometimes demanding people can sometimes lead to the perception that patients when not compliant, are 'the enemy', especially when stress levels are high! The wards are not always healing environments. Along with the possible noise levels and constant activity is the perceived busyness of staff that discourages social interaction, and often discourages the will to ask something. "Oh, they're so busy, I daren't ask" is not an uncommon remark made to me. That can't be good.

Whilst boundaries can be important in care, as a means of helping people to feel secure, there always needs to be a bit of give and take. The recent practice of nurses wearing a red tabard during drug rounds may be seen as admirable in view of mistakes made through distractions regularly encountered during this time. The tabard is easily seen and reads "Do Not Disturb Drug Round in Progress". A boundary that is intended to limit patient intervention for half an hour in order to cut down medication errors seems to make good sense and constitutes good care for that reason. However to the already anxious patient who may need something very important to them like a commode or a painkiller I suspect this kind of perceived stonewalling might turn out to be another nail in the coffin of their self-esteem. The emphasis on nurse concentration might well be missed. Patient vulnerability may well increase because of this well-meaning attempt to improve a service. It confirms the old adage that you can't do right for doing wrong!

Pressure on resources

Cutbacks over the years as with all public services along with technological and pharmaceutical advances have made the NHS a ship caught in a storm. Today arthroscopies such as hips and knees that were only done *in extremis* 30 years ago are now routinely carried out. The same applies to heart bypass operations. All this has been wonderful news to sufferers of course. New drug therapies that are more focused but are very expensive to develop those drugs such as Prednisolone and Interferon are rolled out where funding allows and have very useful results. However it all costs. This could not have been foreseen when the NHS was born nearly 65 years ago. When we add to this the fact of a significantly larger population since 1948 with an increasingly elderly sector, self-induced medical conditions due to drug and alcohol abuse, and the fact that the United Kingdom offers free healthcare to all then funding problems are not surprising. In 1948 with the fallout from two World Wars, the NHS seemed just a godsend to many, particularly to those who had loved ones who came home maimed, disorientated and often requiring some kind of lifetime care. Now old hospital buildings are regularly being replaced by new ones. Yet we still have to discover what the effects of the many Private Finance Initiative builds might be in the future, evidence seems to be emerging that they are bringing pressures on the system.

It is no surprise to see that everything to do with healthcare costs; someone has to pay. The NHS is caught in the horns of a dilemma. Over the years a Post-War idealism has been replaced by practical realism over an institution which was once the envy of other nations but which has become something of a sacred cow as well as a political football in British life. It will be noticed how often the NHS, locally and nationally is in the news. Even sacred cows need water to survive!

Maybe the time has come for the unimaginable; a properly means tested Health Insurance to provide further needed funding for a creaking institution but at the same time a an essential service. With the rising numbers of elderly people who often seem stuck in hospital beds through no fault of their own and the inability of care homes to cope, there is going to be a growing pressure on the Heath Service in the first two decades of the 21st century. Wherever you look at today's hospitals, there is a sense of much being asked of a staff that is shell-shocked with continuous changes to leadership, procedures, targets, employment structures and so on. It is a miracle it succeeds as well as it does.

Perhaps an investment in professionally trained and suitable visitors may add a dimension of empathetic care on the wards to take some expectation away from beleaguered staff. The present Patient Advocacy and Liaison Service may be perceived as taking the 'King's Shilling' in terms of being on the Hospital's side in terms of complaints. Chaplains are growing fewer in number and are always hampered by the misunderstanding from people that their only interest is religious when in fact it is far broader. Something new is needed to add the oil of compassion to the whole service on a larger scale than at present.

We probably know all this. I have no ready answers and my expertise for what it is worth is not in healthcare administration. The next years will show successfully things will be addressed. I shall finish by hoping that the nettle of Bedside Manna will be grasped; that whole people will be recognised by the NHS with *all* their needs, not just the aspects that have "gone wrong". It is simply about giving the person back to the patient, the challenge that Chris Swift gives. Perhaps 'John's' experience highlights what any member of the healthcare team might be faced with in the operating theatre, ward or Accident and Emergency Department. "John was more than a heart muscle, however. He was more than a pump that needed servicing. He was a terrified human being, and his emotional distress was having adverse effect on his medical condition." (**67**) This in my opinion sums it all up. Trauma is everywhere when sickness and accident are, body fixing on its own cannot address this fact.

A woman I once met in cardiology told me that she had a recent bereavement in the family and a pressing Ofsted Inspection at work that really required her presence, particularly as a number of others relied upon her. However she experienced a break-in at home where her computer was stolen with all the materials required for assessment contained in it. They were gone forever. Soon after this she began to experience chest pains. She was very anxious. It was probably not my place to say it but I expressed to her, "If what had happened to you happened to me I think I'd have chest pains too!" I felt I should offer this as a non-medic, as I had personally experienced similar chest pains during a time of particular stress. I knew my thoughts wouldn't be considered particularly authoritative, and all procedures and tests were to follow anyway, and she took my comments as empathetic and not clinical!

Bedside Manna, nurture in a dry place is about taking that *whole* person into the equation. To recognise the trauma in patients' lives would make a difference, it would mean taking more than the body into consideration in the healing dynamic. After 14 years of listening, I *know* there is a huge need. This book has tried to make that point. It attempts to suggest how we might go some of the way to meet it, and get the Health Service and its professionals ask the question; "is this kind of quality care something that the NHS takes seriously alongside the temptation simply to treat persons and not only symptoms because of the financial stringencies of the NHS in the 21st Century; and will funding or at least a more comprehensive education of holistic care be provided to develop it?"

29

FAITH AND PRACTICE

Religion can play an important role in people's lives. It can give them a place of belonging, a sense of meaning, a direction in life and hope. When illness strikes, a sense of God can enable people to place their present and future in a higher power. On these themes are scores of variations. To feel 'held' or borne up on the prayers of others, is a feeling many have told me about on the wards. In short religion gives people connection. When I speak of religion I do not mean the thinly disguised tribalism that considers all those outside its fold as lesser beings, but that movement of people's hearts which uplifts and enriches the adherent in recognition of a higher power, and for whom love of neighbor is paramount.

Some people particularly from the Christian tradition may be a little dismayed that this book is not as overtly *Christian* as they would expect. This book is not about presenting the Christian faith to patients. The fact that a chaplain is writing it may invite the response among some people " well, that's what they do, isn't it?" Actually, within the whole line up of church ministries there are others more gifted to present the faith to the world. If we did that in a hospital setting it would be both invasive and manipulative, two things you simply do not with vulnerable people in the position of being a captive audience. Spiritual care requires sensitivity to the primary needs of ill people. Whilst we do not shy away from discussing matters of faith, even controversial ones with those who invite the conversation, introducing the subject is not what we do. As St Francis of Assisi is reputed to have said " Preach the Gospel at all times and where necessary use words." Our ministry is largely wordless from that point of view. The care we show for others, if that doesn't sound too smug, should be demonstration enough of where we are coming from. Routinely though, chaplains meet the religious needs of patients with conversation, prayer and bringing Holy Communion and anointing with oil for healing to the bedside, as well as holding services in the Chapel. Muslim chaplains meet prayer and other religious needs within their own faith community.

Perhaps the same people who imagine that we should be more proactively faith promoting may have the expectation that this text will be punctuated by Biblical quotations, references to God, Jesus and the Holy Spirit. They might expect to see the role of the whole Church emphasised more as a body whose role it is to comfort the afflicted. My disclaimer here is that although I am an ordained Church of England priest, I also recognise that so many of the primary aims in spiritual care are driven by an approach congenial to the mind and attitude of Jesus as we are introduced to it in the Gospels. In one of the Gospels the visiting of the sick is likened to caring for Jesus himself, "I was sick and you looked after me." **(68)** In this passage Jesus is shown as representing the face of the poor, marginalised and vulnerable in society. This would also aptly describe the sick. It is also observable that the same high aims are shared by other faith traditions as well as many "people of goodwill". I can certainly live with that. As you read on, perhaps you may see the many connections with the Biblical tradition woven into the text, but not necessarily painted in bold colours. Spiritual carers will not always be card carrying followers of a particular religious tradition. Overall, I personally believe that the recognisable stamp of the Suffering Servant runs through the previous pages. "He was despised and rejected by men, a man of sorrows and familiar with suffering, like one from whom men hide their faces." **(69)** This statement is hardly a far cry from the experience of the chronically ill.

While it is inevitable that any account of the more inner aspects of the patient experience written by a chaplain will allude to religious and spiritual matters, I have tried to keep them to a minimum to retain the attention of people for whom these things may not be relevant to their own lives. I have had to explore spiritual care so far (as opposed to religious care) as it is an inescapable factor which presents itself when our deeper selves cry out at that moment when meaning, purpose and value seem to evaporate in the face of illness and the like. I have largely dealt with this in Chapter 5, where I also reference some valuable research that points to the benefits faith confers upon people in relation to their journey through ill health.

You will find that I have drawn upon varied sources to illustrate what I have tried to say, both from the sacred and secular, spiritual and contemporary news sources. Inevitably my references will show the reader where I am coming from. What feeds me may also feed others, irrespective of the brand label of the source.

Secular wisdom and religious and spiritual insights are never too distant from each other.

We borrow from all sources that in difficult times carry meaning for us. I have mentioned the Psalms before as a body of reflection that echo recognisable feelings that we all experience during the traumas experienced while we are in hospital and exiled from the world we know. We wrestle; the Psalmist wrestles.

Similarly many parts of the Bible can bring uplift, which I can testify to, even among the non 'faith card carrying' community. The thoughtful parables and punchy one liners of Jesus still have the effect of pushing those buttons of insight that give hope and meaning in the midst of crisis. Most especially his treatment of compassion in everyday life gives a pointer to how the care in healthcare might ideally be managed. A tall order maybe, but if we reach for the stars we might finish up with a higher standard than before. Specifically the parable of the Good Samaritan highlights the tension between instinctive compassion and professionalism; something the NHS grapples with perennially.

IS COMPASSION ONLY AN OPTIONAL EXTRA FOR THE NHS?

The term 'Good Samaritan' is regularly used by people in describing a person who does another a good turn, but it is so much more than that. As a springboard for the parable Jesus is asked by a good living upright and religious man how he can improve on his life. Jesus first informs him of the distillation of the Mosaic Law that he should love God and his neighbour *as himself.* The last phrase is significant, because this man for all his credibility still feels that he's not there yet.

173

Jesus responds to his reply "And who is my neighbour" by telling a story of a man who is mugged, beaten up and left for dead in the road.

Jesus further describes how two characters pass this way, squint at the bloodied body and move on quickly. They are both high profile religious figures in the Palestine of the day, a priest and a Levite (a helper in Temple duties). *Professionals*, if you like. Both had duties in the Temple, and to be in contact with a dead body, or so they thought, would render them contaminated therefore impure for their work. They were not bad people, but they made their choices according to what governed their lives.

The Samaritan, on the other hand, was a mixed-race, theologically doubtful character and looked down on as far as contemporary Judaism was concerned. But he just couldn't help himself. His heart overcame his theology and he responded to this beaten up victim of crime. He was compassionate. He felt a fellow empathetic suffering with this poor unfortunate. He offered care and basic first aid. He then decided on appropriate follow up journeying with the victim to an inn where he set him up with longer provision for his recovery. It didn't stop there, the Samaritan offered that if expenses were to exceed what he has already paid, then he would be back to pay the balance. Presumably the landlord knew him for who he was and readily agreed.

The point that is being made here is that it is fine to be holy and keep your rules of purity, but we are in theory a *neighbour* to everyone, whether they are despised, looking half dead or whatever. In terms of the Jewish purity codes, according to Jesus, compassion out trumps religious observance if the wellbeing of another is threatened. The Samaritan was led by his heart so he instinctively responded to the man's need. He had positive self-esteem (he loved himself) unlike the young man who enquired who his neighbour was with Jesus, whom he knew to have *something* he didn't. Interestingly this parable only appears in Luke's Gospel; tradition having it that the author was both an outsider Gentile and a doctor! (70) Jesus's final words to his enquirer were "Go and do likewise". A cue perhaps for the NHS!

RELIGIOUS NEEDS AND BOUNDARIES

The NHS is committed to respond to the religious needs of patients in the best way they can. I have mentioned in Chapter 13 how Muslims can feel fragile if their cultural and religious needs are ignored. It can lead to some anxiety, and an erosion of safety and familiarity which we all need when faced with the unusual. If prayer cannot be easily performed in the appropriate way, it may well affect the Muslim patient's peace of mind.

A Muslim chaplain or local Imam can reassure a person that they do not have to face Mecca as they pray in bed, or even prostrate themselves. What is not possible in hospital is simply not possible but permitted in their faith because of the unusual circumstances. If people don't know that, they may continue to get caught in a cycle of guilt and confusion that may run counter to the healing process.

Experience over the years has shown me that when human need is extreme boundaries are more easily crossed. I can remember being called in to offer prayers for a dying Hindu man, whose family appeared fully confident that I could do what was required in the circumstances. On another occasion I was asked to take the funeral of a small baby whose parents were Muslim. The mother was White British and had married a Muslim man and converted. I talked through the delicacy of the situation with them, but they were happy to go ahead. I dipped into over the Koran and the Wisdom literature of the Bible to draw out what would bring comfort. It passed off perfectly well.

There was another occasion when a Roman Catholic family has simply asked for the chaplain on duty to say prayers over a dying relative, as they were accepting that someone on hand might do as well as a priest whom they had to 'dig out' from what other pressing duties he might have. I remember another two occasions; one where no amount of phoning about could raise a Roman Catholic chaplain or local priest. This went on for hours and it was an anxiety for the family. Then like the proverbial buses, three turned up at the same time! The other was when a patient I knew died on the ward and I was rung up to summon a suitable spiritual caregiver from their own denomination. No one turned up, and this went on all morning. I knew also that the ward staff were anxious to have the bed. We have to observe protocols, but it this situation was getting more and more trying. The patient, whom I had visited the day before for about the third time was very dead and getting very cold. In a moment of inspiration, I thought commonsense must prevail, so I told the staff someone was coming in (after five hours) but not that it was me. I said the prayers and kept very *schtum* - forever. I am not certain that he would have taken exception but . . . boundaries sometimes have to be crossed in extreme cases.

Because this chapter deals with the religious side of things, this is a moment to express some sadness. Some of the most difficult people to support in my experience have been what I would describe as very keen, even extreme Christians. I found that in many cases an iron-clad belief was simply a mask for denial. I have witnessed a number of these people die still holding on to the notion that their illness was a test; that God would heal them miraculously; and that they were in hospital to share their faith with other patients and staff. They failed to see that being human is not in opposition to having faith and that vulnerability in the face of trials and difficulties is not denying what they believe. Thankfully meeting these people was not an everyday encounter, and most people we did meet seemed to take the rough with the smooth without any need to make themselves out to be riding above it all.

AN INVENTORY OF CHAPLAINCY INTERVENTIONS

Generally chaplaincy was not enlisted in the NHS as a provision to convert people or indeed espouse any particular faith tradition to the unwary patient. As our chaplaincy was both inter-denominational and multifaith we had most bases covered anyway. Whilst many approaches were taken to patient support from their religious point of view, what we could offer was a non-judgmental listening ear, a link with local faith traditions, a place of quiet and worship. There were times when we were asked to set up a Humanist funeral or make provision for other spiritual caregivers from Jewish and Buddhist traditions as well as Pagan upon request. We made routine ward visits and crisis visiting when ward staff, relatives or local church leaders alerted us. From time to time we prayed with people when asked, provided spiritual reading matter, and used anointing with oil and prayers for the dying from time to time, often on call-outs in the night. On one occasion we anointed an elderly clergyperson at his request, and with much trepidation we did it, only to find he went into almost immediate remission and wrote to us thanking us . . . "o ye of little faith!"

Some of these have been mentioned in passing, but as chaplains we conducted funerals, blessed babies upon birth and after neonatal death, supported parents and were part of the hospital Trust and helped with funerals and memorial services related to staff. We did Sunday Services, marriages, christenings when a patient was unlikely to survive. It was a privilege, and I hope we never took advantage of our position. When Princess Diana died and the events of 9/11 required an institutional response we opened a Book of Condolence in the Chapel. We also tried to support seasonal moments for patients, particularly in rehabilitation as I have mentioned, primarily to create an *at-home* atmosphere for them in hospital. As this may convey, chaplains do have to be Jack and Jaquelines of-all-trades.

In trying to provide familiarity both emotionally and spiritually for patients, sometimes the opposite was happening to us chaplains at the same time. The effect of journeying with patients and staff on me personally over the years was that of creating *dis-comfort zones* that I had not encountered in parish ministry. There were situations that fazed me, pain I found hard to reconcile with a loving God, and hassles that I wish I could have been free from. No; hospitals are real life, and chaplains are not immune from that. I believe these things can only be for the good. They certainly kept me on a growing edge and enabled me to avoid the pitfall of complacency. Often I was truly admiring of the faith and fortitude of others who supported patients better than I could, through thick and thin.

30

THE HEALERS

To conclude, the point has been made that the holistic and spiritual care needed by people in hospital and ill health, can be provided by a whole range of people. It is an art to be learned, not a science to be applied. Because it is emotionally costly and draining it is too often avoided on the pretext of professional detachment. This really amounts to a rationing of quality time with people who need it.

This care goes beyond the medical, vital as it is, and enlivens the individual to find their lives again. It enables resilience to face another day with hope. A heartening story is told by Harold Kushner as he describes a family disrupted by the practical consequences of an unexpected death, and the general onset of old age disadvantaged by this loss of support. An elderly widow lived with her son in his fifties who saw to her care and practical needs, whilst her other sons had moved away from the region. The son who was carer died of a heart attack and the distraught woman had lost everything at a stroke. The other sons stepped in and were looking to find a nursing home after their mother grew depressed and confused and could not find the strength for housework and cooking.

Among the homes they visited was one where this woman's seventy-something cousin was living. Far from recommending his living situation, he found much to find fault with both with the food and the staff. It did not look at all encouraging. Out of the blue one of the staff (they could not remember quite *who* it was) had the idea that the cousin left the nursing home and moved in with the widow. As the family discovered, the results were startling. Whether we put this inspirational thought down to practical or holistic or spiritual care, it nonetheless took wisdom, intuition and the best interests of both parties into account; and moreover, worked. Kushner describes the results: "Like a parched plant that people begin to water, the widow seemed to grow younger and healthier daily. Having someone to share her life with, someone who needed her, gave her back her reasons for living. She had been on the verge of dying of loneliness, and now she had reasons to get up in the morning and look forward to the new day." (71)

The good news is that *all* who support patients, whether clinicians, managers, chaplains, porters and domestic staff, family and local social or church friends are *part* of the healing team, which this following poem brings out. Some may do it naturally, others may need quite a lot of time and training. The qualification is that of being a fellow human being, like the Good Samaritan, who saw the mugged man's need and did not pass by, but did what he could because it sprang from the heart. It costs, but doesn't everything we consider worthwhile? Long may the Bedside Manna distributors bring refreshment and nurture to those in the desert of ill health. May the Health Service take heed with a more robust recognition and provision for *what lies within.*

THE HEALERS

He placed the card upon the shelf; the girl, her sightless eyes,
Would never see the love it brought and cry with brief surprise.
She sat in silence, while the grief was gripping at her soul;
Her mother fighting for each breath, too desperate to console.

The man sat slumped behind the screens, restraining needs to yell;
While doctors muffled, shuffled feet and wondered what to tell.
The wife of youth and now of age pushed him round the grounds,
The dreams of their retirement now a wreck of mocking sounds.

The chaplain felt the pain around of all that "might have been"
Wondering often how to help; or else to leave the scene.
We care for patients in their beds, relieved to see them leave,
But often fail to notice those who care and hope and grieve.

Spare a moment's thought or prayer, for those who stand and wait,
Those who yearn, the ones who learn to share and bear the weight.

Be gentle with the mother who, for want of tears to weep
Stays by the bed of her dear son a sleepless watch to keep.

Remember all love's bonds that get so tangled in life's storms;
The loss that draws the wayward heart, and helps strong ties to form.
Remember that the human heart may, weaken, wander, wane;
But also waken, pulse and fly; aroused by others' pain.

The ones who walk the corridors, who sit in wards and yearn,
Discover sweeter springs of care well up from what they learn.
The rhythms that immerse their lives, the ups and downs they feel,
Go to form those pearls inside, and healing gifts reveal.

NOTES

1) World Health Organisation. Definition of Health approved by the 52nd World Health Assembly 1999.

2) Your Guide to the NHS. Department of Health 2011

3) Pemberton M. Finger on the Pulse Daily Telegraph 21 January 2011

4) Rt Rev Herbert C. The Lord Bishop of St Albans; The Palliative Care Bill. Second Reading. House of Lords Debates. 23rd February 2007

5) Jennings K. NHS 'Customer Service' a Priority. BBC News www. bbc.co.uk Health 21st June 2007

6) Odone C. Mail on Line. www.dailymail.co.uk/femail/article 1023505 1st June 2008

7) Youngson R. Compassion in Healthcare. NHS Futures Debate. May 2008

8) Davis C. The Temptations of Religion. Hodder and Stoughton 1973

9) Swift C. Meeting Change with Good Faith. Amicus Health. Spring 2007

10) Marcus Borg. The Heart of Christianity. Harper SanFrancisco 2003

11) Leighty J. Studer Group. Studer Nursing Spectrum. 20th November 2006

12) Armstrong L. It's Not About The Bike. Berkley Books. 2001

13) Murray RB. Zentner JP. Nursing Concepts for Health Promotion. Prentice Hall. London

14) Johnston D. Mayers CA. Response. In Mayers CA. letters page, British Journal of Occupational Therapy 67 (6) 2004

15) Persaud R. Thank God for your Good Health. News Review. The Sunday Times. June 4th 2000

16) Koenig HG. Larsen DB. Spirituality: a review of Occupational Therapy. British Journal of Occupational Therapy 68 (9) 2005

17) Galloway K. Getting Personal. SPCK. 1995

18) Cressey R. Winbolt-Lewis M. The Forgotten Heart of Care. Journal of Accident and Emergency Nursing. 2000(8)

19) McSherry W. Nurses Perception of Spirituality and Spiritual Care. Nursing Standard 13 (4) 1998

20) St Mark's Gospel. Chapter 1 verses 40-44

21) Price JL. Stevens HO. Labarre MC. Journal of Psychosocial Nursing. Vol 33 (12) 1995

22) Holistic and Spiritual Care Policy. Chaplaincy: Mid Yorkshire Hospitals NHS

Trust. revised June 2010

23) Youngson R. Compassion in Healthcare. NHS Futures Debate. May 2008

24) Taylor JV. The Go Between God. SCMPress 1972

25) Nouwen H. The Wounded Healer. Image Books 1979

26) Borg M. The Heart of Christianity. HarperSanFrancisco 2003

27) Dalal I. Nursing Standard. Vol 22 (4) 3rd October 2007

28) Cassidy S. Good Friday People. Darton, Longman & Todd 1991

29) Cassidy S. Light from the Dark Valley. Darton, Longman & Todd 1994

30) Khan Q. A Day in the Life. Volume 10 issue 4 November 2006 Pavilion Journals (Brighton) Ltd

31) Jung C. The Symbolic Life: Miscellaneous Writings. The Collected Works Vol 18. Routledge and Kegan Paul 1956/1977

32) Tuckwell G Flagg D. A Question of Healing. Harper Collins. London 1995

33) Moltmann J. Theology and Joy. SCM Press 1973

34) Williams HHA. The True Resurrection. Mitchell and Beasley 1972

35) Chown A. The Lessons that Cancer Taught me. Daily Telegraph October 26th 2004

36) NICE Guidance on Cancer Care: Improving Supporting and Palliative Care for Adults with Cancer. Spiritual Support Services 2004

37) Mann I. A Double Thirst. Darton, Longman & Todd. 2001.

38) Psalm 22. Verses 1-2. New International Version

39) Moir J. Moir on Wednesday. Daily Telegraph. 29th May 2007

40) Odone C. I Refused to let my Father Die. Daily Telegraph. October 18th 2010

41) Winterman D. How to live, by the dying. BBC News. www. bbc.co.uk Magazine 3rd January 2008

42) Emerson RW. Journals. 1821 cited by Speck P. in Being There SPCK Press 1988

43) Stress Link to Heart Disease BBC News. www.bbc.co.uk Health 21st November 2002.

44) Stress Link to Chronic Fatigue BBC News. www. bbc.co.uk Health 30th November 2002

45) Stress 'Hinders Healing Process' BBC News. www.bbc.co.uk Health 5th December 2005

46) Stress Ages Immune System. BBC News. www. bbc.co.uk. Health 5th July 2003

47) Kelly L. Listening to patients: a lifetime perspective from Ian McWhinney.

CJRM (3) 1998

48) Youngson R. Compassion in Healthcare. NHS Futures Debate. May 2008

49) Rogers, C. On Becoming a Person. Boston: Houghton Mifflin. 1961.

50) Nouwen H. Reaching Out Collins/Fount 1988

51) Stoter D. Spiritual Aspects of Healthcare. Mosby 1995.

52) Perry B. Influence of Nurse Gender on the use of silence, touch and humour. International Journal of Palliative Medicine. Vol 2 2 (1) 1996

53) Ryan S. BBC Man's Despair at Losing Second Child. The Daily Telegraph. May 3rd 2001

54) Youngson R. Compassion in Healthcare. NHS Futures Debate. May 2008

55) Elisabeth Kubler-Ross. On Death and Dying. Routledge 1995

56) Tuckwell G.and Flagg D. A Question of Healing. Harper/Collins 1995

57) Lawrence DH. Poem "Healing" quoted in Faith, Spirituality and Music Therapy Journal of Healthcare Chaplains Vol 5 (2) 2004

58) A Time to Heal. A Contribution towards the Ministry of Healing Church of England Church House Publishing 2000

59) www.teenagecancertrust.org/who-we-are/media-centre/press-release/jason-manford 30th June 2011

60) Davies J. Health Service Journal. 15th July 2004

61) Nouwen H. Reaching Out. Collins/Fount 1988

62) Neuburger J. The Spiritual Challenge of Health Care. ed. Cobb M. Robshaw V. Churchill Livingstone 1998

63) Campbell AV. Paid to Care? SPCK Publishing 1988

64) Odone C. I Refused to let my Father Die. Daily Telegraph October 18th 2010

65) Warner F. A Gentle Dying Hay House 2008 also www.soulmidwives.co.uk

66) Parkinson F. Coping with Post-Trauma Stress. Sheldon Press. 2000

67) Di Matteo MR. The Psychology of Health, Illness and Medical Care. Brooks/Cole Publishing Company 1991

68) St Matthew's Gospel. Chapter 25 verses 34-40. New International Version.

69) Isaiah. Chapter 53 verse 3. New International Version.

70) Luke's Gospel. Chapter 10 Verses 25-37 New International Version

71) Kushner H. Who needs God? Simon & Schuster NY (Fireside) 2002

ACKNOWLEDGMENTS

I want to thank Roger Cressey who took the risk of appointing me in 1996 to work alongside him in patient and staff support and developing the understanding of spiritual care in Pinderfields Hospital, as it then was. He allowed me to share in the writing of several papers on spiritual care and thus left me a sound legacy to build upon.

I also acknowledge my colleagues in Chaplaincy, both Christian and Muslim whole and part-time who have offered support, friendship and the pearl of mutual peer evaluation. I must mention Mary Gaskell, John Arnold, Martin Parrott, John Taylor and Jonathan Sharp. None of this would happen of course without the hard working staff and many patients who allowed me to enter their lives, sometimes briefly, but who have helped to create this book. On patient confidentiality, my disclaimer is that names, circumstances and certain details have been altered to protect identification. Every effort has been made to protect the identities of those mentioned in the above pages, except where express permission has been granted. In fact some episodes happened so long ago I should not be able to put a name to a pseudonym myself!

I want to acknowledge Sue Campbell, the Chair of the Trust Board in the early years for her interest and encouragement, and to Julia Squire Chief Executive of the Mid Yorkshire NHS Trust latterly, who took a supportive interest in chaplaincy. I am grateful to the late Mary Lowe and Anne Kennedy who shepherded us wisely on the path of chaplaincy modernisation. I am indebted to all my Line Managers and colleagues in the various Directorates that embraced that Cinderella of the NHS - chaplaincy! Special acknowledgement is due also to Geoff Naylor who contributed his wisdom in laborious readings and editing of this text, and my mother Joycie, who with the strength available to her in her 95 year, aided me over the finishing line.

Finally I am only too aware of the many sacrifices made by my family because of the chaplain in the family, particularly by my wife Sue. On-call duties often meant not being able to do things that we should have liked, and rapidly having to change plans when the pager went off. Thank you for your forbearance.

ABOUT THE AUTHOR

Martin Winbolt-Lewis has led a varied life ranging from Olympic athlete to minicab driver; Guinness Book of Records editorial assistant to university journalist, and BBC research worker to house warden of an international students club in London. From 1975, ordained in the Church of England, he served in several parishes before becoming a chaplain in 1996 in a West Yorkshire NHS Trust which grew from one to three hospitals. Having retired in 2011 he is involved now with in the Ripon & Leeds Diocese in spiritual direction and learning disabilities. Martin enjoys sport, walking, travel, reading, crosswords and music of all kinds. He is a published poet and lives with his wife Sue in Yorkshire. They have four children and are also grandparents.

Lightning Source UK Ltd.
Milton Keynes UK
UKOW032133240613

212751UK00023B/1461/P